RELAXERCISE

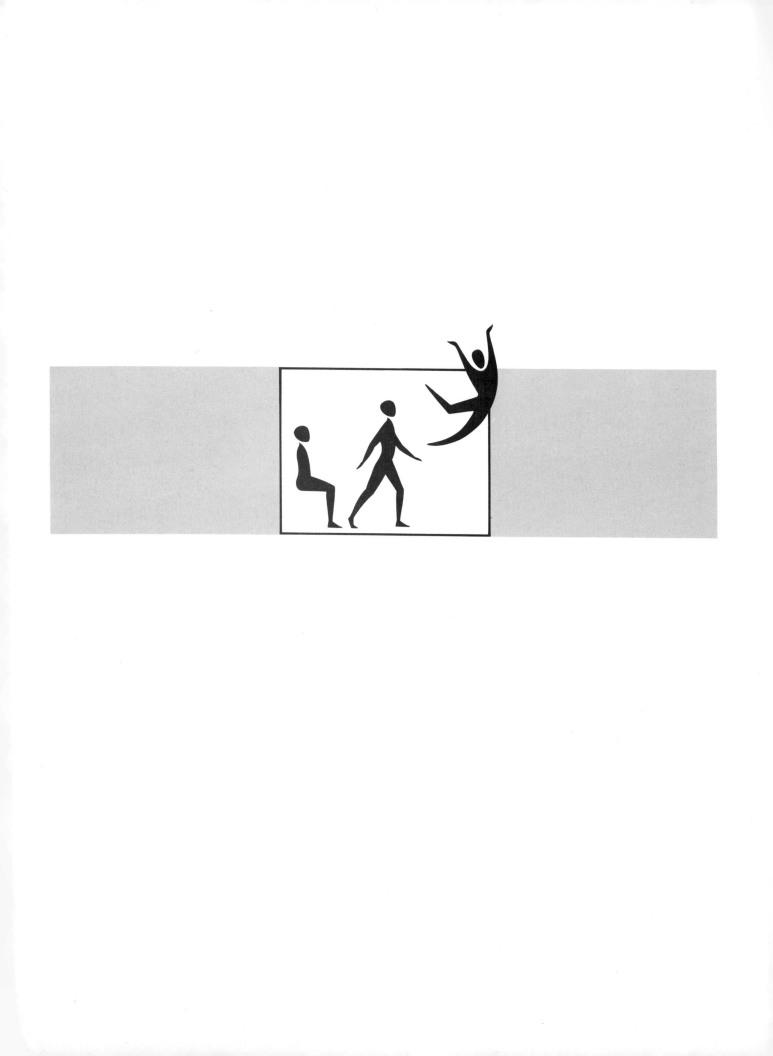

RELAXERCISE

THE EASY NEW WAY
TO HEALTH & FITNESS

DAVID ZEMACH-BERSIN

KAETHE ZEMACH-BERSIN

MARK REESE

1817

Harper & Row, Publishers, San Francisco

New York, Grand Rapids, Philadelphia, St. Louis
London, Singapore, Sydney, Tokyo, Toronto

NOTE

Though thousands of people have benefited from doing Relaxercise exercises, we cannot anticipate the special needs, limitations, and responses of every individual. The information contained in this book is not intended for the purpose of diagnosing or as a substitute for medical treatment. Consult your doctor before beginning this or any other exercise program. We cannot and do not offer any warranty of the effectiveness of the exercises. Responsibility for the results of the exercises is necessarily the reader's.

If you have any questions, you may communicate with the authors by writing to Sensory Motor Learning Systems, P.O. Box 5674, Berkeley, California, 94705.

Photo of Dr. Feldenkrais © Bonnie Freer
All other photos © Richard Blair
Illustrations © Kaethe Zemach-Bersin

FIRST EDITION

Library of Congress Cataloging-in-Publication Data

Zemach-Bersin, David.
    Relaxercise: the new way to feel good.

      Bibliography: p.
    1. Exercise.   2. Motor ability.   3. Mind and body.
I. Zemach-Bersin, Kaethe. II. Reese, Mark. III. Title.
RA781.Z46 1989   613.7'1   89-45242
ISBN 0-06-250992-6

90 91 92 93 94 K.P. 10 9 8 7 6 5 4 3 2 1

In Honor of
Moshe Feldenkrais, D.Sc.
1904–1984

for
Doris Falender
1928–1989
whose friendship and encouragement
helped make the impossible, possible.

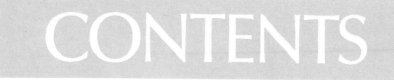

CONTENTS

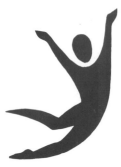

1. EASY FLEXIBILITY   21

Learn how to improve your flexibility and freedom of movement by as much as 100%!

2. LOW BACK COMFORT   35

Give yourself immediate relief and find a way to end chronic low back tension.

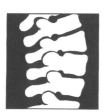

3. A HEALTHY SPINE   47

Restore the health and flexibility of your spine and counteract the effects of sedentary living.

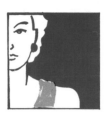

4. RELAXED SHOULDERS   57

Learn how to eliminate tension and discomfort from the most vulnerable part of your body while improving your range of motion.

5. YOUR POWER CENTER   71

Mobilize the most powerful muscles of your body to improve your ease of movement and posture.

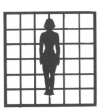
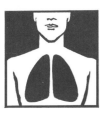
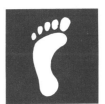
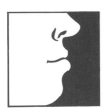
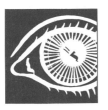
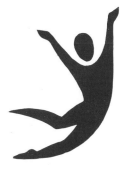

PREFACE

For the last fifteen years, Dr. Mark Reese and I have been helping people to find solutions to their physical problems, pains and disabilities. We've found that almost all men and women reach adulthood without the benefit of some essential information about how their body works. Without an understanding of the basic physical and structural laws that govern our body, we unwittingly develop neuromuscular habits which are physically stressful and increase our vulnerability to injury. As a consequence, we eventually suffer from an infinite variety of physical problems from back-ache, headache, neck and shoulder pain, to loss of flexibility, tension and fatigue. These problems are **not** a necessary part of either modern life or getting older.

It's never too late to learn and change. We've found that 95% of our client's physical complaints are easy to remedy, quick to improve and can ultimately be avoided. Learning a few simple principles of healthy body usage can help us to maintain our body's flexibility and comfort throughout our entire life, prevent aches and pains, and enable us to heal rapidly when injuries do occur.

We have worked hard to create a book which will give you both the information and the means to attain a comfortable, pain-free and healthy body. We hope you will enjoy the exercises and illustrations, and find this new, extraordinary approach to a healthy body exciting and refreshing. Welcome to **Relaxercise**.

David Zemach-Bersin
Berkeley, California

FOREWORD

by Harold Bloomfield, M.D.

How many times have you tried to force yourself to start exercising regularly and take more time for relaxation? And how many times have you found that the system you tried didn't work or helped only for a short while? Most conventional exercise systems are based on the assumption that the human body is a machine that can be forced to work by hammering, twisting, oiling, and kicking. But the body is not a machine; it is an enormously complex living system.

Health and fitness isn't just a matter of finding the "right technique" and adjusting the body to run smoothly. Human beings aren't sports cars in need of a good tune-up. Something more is required: a new vision of the fully functioning person, a new model of health and fitness.

The creation of this new vision is an enormous task that has been going on in many universities and institutions all over the world for the last twenty years. Dr. Moshe Feldenkrais, on whose work **Relaxercise** is based, was one of the great pioneers of this new vision of health.

Human beings are created with an unlimited capacity for growth. Unfortunately, most of us use but 5 to 10 percent of our intellectual, emotional, and physical capacity. **Relaxercise** will help to awaken your capacity for improved health and well-being so you can begin to create the life you really want.

Most fitness books and health educators put forward the antiquated idea that achieving health and flexibility is an arduous task that requires considerable time, self-denial, and sometimes even pain. **Relaxercise** demonstrates that this isn't true; it provides, instead, a step-by-step program which utilizes the extraordinary natural abilities of your brain to improve the health of your body. Rather than exhort you to follow punishing regimens of stretching and exercise, **Relaxercise** will show you how to effortlessly tap your deepest capacities for fitness and health.

Relaxercise will show you how to achieve a state of fitness and well-being that will afford greater enjoyment of living. You will learn how to slow the aging process. You will learn how to increase your flexibility, your coordination and your grace of movement. You will improve your posture. Finally, you will learn to look better and feel better, and with each succeeding year look forward to further rewards from living.

This book can be instrumental in helping you to achieve your full measure of health and vitality. **Relaxercise** is a quantum leap in the discovery and creation of practical techniques for realizing health and fitness. **Relaxercise** is superb! It is the best how-to book I have read for improving your body's flexibility, relaxation, posture, vitality and comfort. Use it please!

ACKNOWLEDGMENTS

We wish to thank everyone who helped make this book possible. Our special thanks to Chuck Moshontz, for his help in the creation of Relaxercise. We are indebted to him for his commitment, contribution, and friendship. We also wish to thank: Debbie Ostrow and Heidi Zemach for their long hours of typing, Doris Worthington for her research skills, Fred Falender for his support and belief in Relaxercise, Bernard Scheier at Harper & Row for his support and patience, Terri Goff for her help and editorial skills, John Loudon for his commitment to this book as it grew beyond its original scope, Irene Imfeld for her contribution to the design of Relaxercise, Eileen Vollowitz of Back Design, Inc., for her critical reading of Part 3, Gaby Yaron, Mia Segal, Ruthy Alon and Yochanon Rywerant for their inspired teaching, Alisa Colloms and Rebecca Zemach for their vital assistance, Jed Appelman and Elizabeth Beringer for their steadfast friendship through the endless months of writing, Margot Zemach for her extraordinary grace, and thanks to our families, Donna, Nathan, and Filip Ray-Reese, Cybele Lerman, and Ariella and Talya Zemach-Bersin for their love and patience. This book is as much theirs as it is ours.

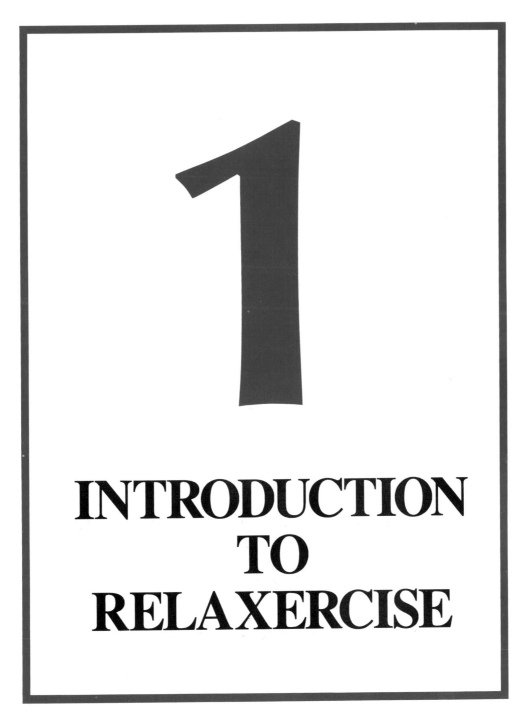

1

INTRODUCTION TO RELAXERCISE

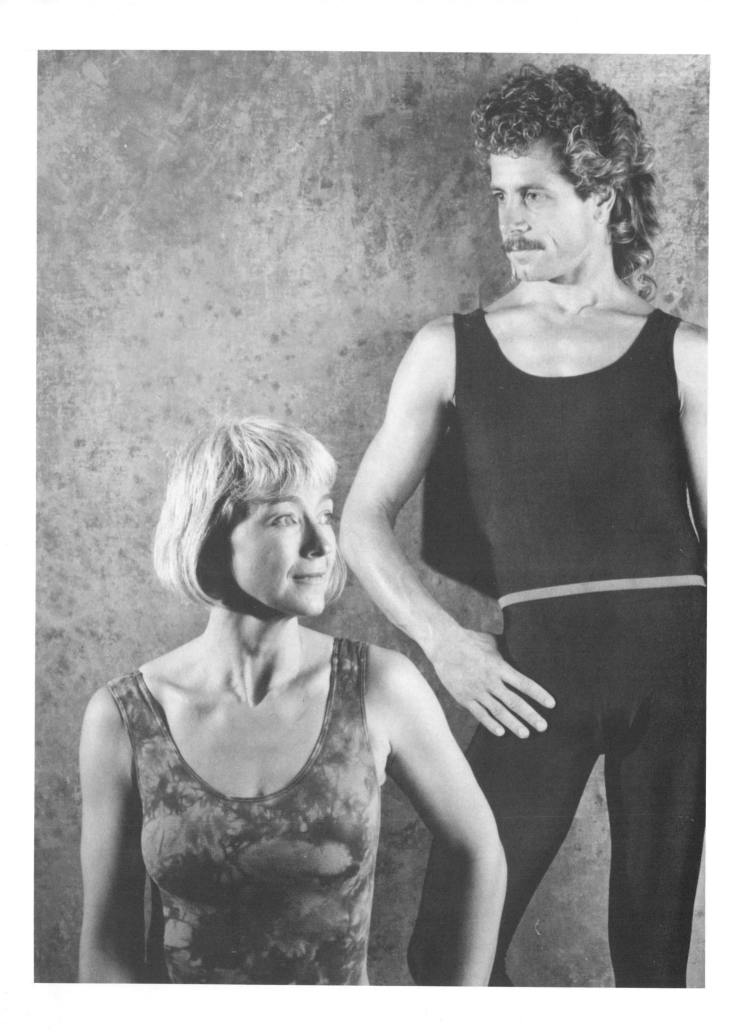

Rē·lax'er·cīse

1. Quick relief from aches and pains. **2.** Immediate improvement in flexibility and posture. **3.** Freedom and ease of movement. **4.** Effective stress reduction. **5.** A great way to feel better!

Like most of us, you are probably looking for an easy and effective way to maintain your physical health and feel better.

Do you suffer nagging aches and pains? Do you often feel tense or stiff? Are you troubled by recurring neck, shoulder, or back problems? Do you notice your ease of movement becoming restricted and your physical vitality diminishing as you grow older? Or are you simply looking for effective ways to maintain your health and youthfulness?

Relaxercise is an extraordinary form of exercise. Scientific breakthroughs in neurophysiology and neuropsychology have revealed that there is a powerful connection between your brain and body and that your brain is capable of improving your body's health and well-being. By harnessing the natural power of your brain, Relaxercise is able to bring your body remarkable benefits that have never before been possible with other exercise systems.

Relaxercise exercises are easy to do. They involve hardly any muscular effort, are safe and effective, and take only fifteen to thirty minutes to do. Best of all, the results and rewards are immediate. With Relaxercise you can begin to feel better right away!

Enjoy the difference!

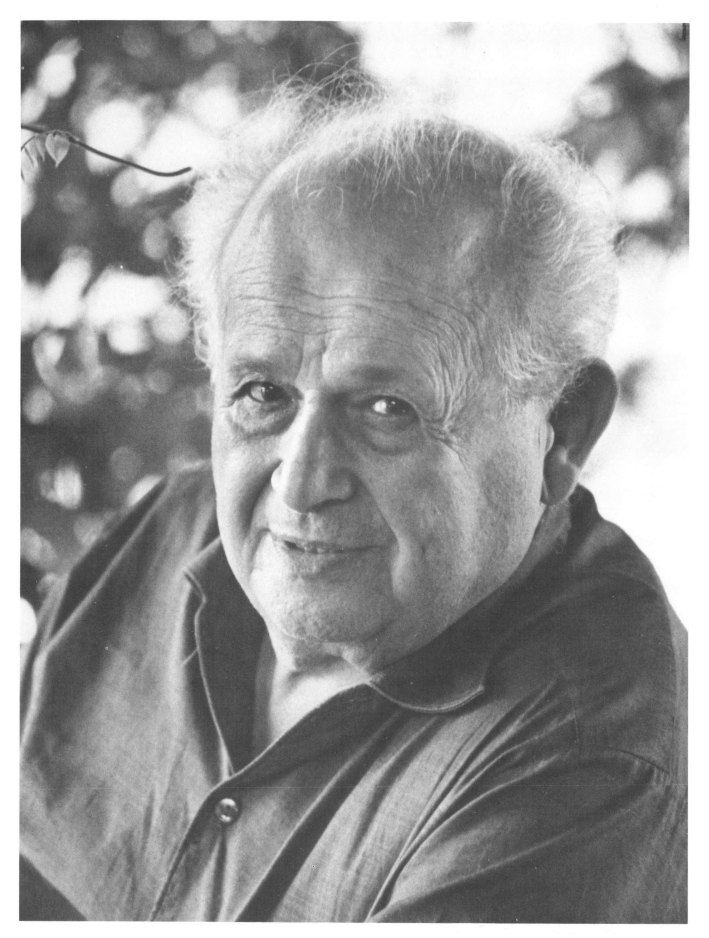

Dr. Moshe Feldenkrais

THE HISTORY OF RELAXERCISE

In 1942, Dr. Moshe Feldenkrais, a brilliant and respected physicist working in London, faced one of the most critical challenges of his lifetime. Because he had suffered a series of sports-related knee injuries, he was now painfully crippled. He was confronted with the possibility that he might have to spend the rest of his life using either crutches or a wheelchair. The medical specialists had given him a disheartening prognosis. In their estimation, there was a 50 percent chance that surgery could repair his knees. But they warned that if the surgery failed, it could drastically reduce his chances of ever being able to walk again. He had to decide: Should he undergo the surgery—or was the risk too great? Might there be other solutions?

Feldenkrais approached his unenviable dilemma with characteristic determination and a special understanding of both the human body and contemporary science. He had been the first European to receive a black belt in the Japanese martial art of judo and had written five definitive books on its technique and theory. As a physicist, Feldenkrais was accustomed to solving problems that had tested the brightest minds of his generation. For many years he had been a close associate of French Nobel laureate physicist Frederic Joliet-Curie. Together they had conducted some of the very first experiments in atomic research. Could Feldenkrais apply his knowledge of physics and the human body to finding a way to regain the use of his legs?

Feldenkrais chose *not* to undergo the proposed surgery. Instead, he began to study neurology, anatomy, biomechanics, and human movement development. He knew that in order to walk again, he would have to find a way to create new neurological connections between his nervous system and his muscles. After two years of research and experimentation, Feldenkrais emerged victorious. He succeeded in completely restoring his ability to walk. Feldenkrais had developed a way to improve his body by *activating the natural power of his brain and nervous system.*

Inspired by his personal success, Feldenkrais continued to explore the profound link between the brain and the body, and developed hundreds of unique exercises designed to access the movement learning centers of the brain. Feldenkrais tested his new ideas with his friends and colleagues. He treated their aches and pains, muscle and joint problems, and even debilitating neurological conditions. One after another, their symptoms disappeared. It was obvious that Feldenkrais had discovered an extraordinary new approach to physical improvement.

In 1949, Feldenkrais published his theories about the relationship between human movement and the nervous system in *Body and Mature Behavior*, a book still widely read. The following year, he became a professor of physics at the famed Weismann Institute in Israel, while continuing to apply and refine his unique neuromuscular exercises. By 1954, there was such a great demand for his new knowledge and skill that he decided to leave physics and dedicate himself to helping others improve their health.

Soon people from all over Europe were traveling to Feldenkrais's popular clinic and classes in Tel-Aviv. His classes were attended not only by people suffering from physical problems but also by musicians, athletes, dancers, and thousands of other people from every walk of life. In 1972, Feldenkrais was invited to the United States to present his work at health institutions and universities. The response was overwhelming, and for the next decade, he spent part of each year in the United States teaching and lecturing.

Before he died in 1984, at the age of eighty, Feldenkrais trained a small group of practitioners to continue his work and make it available to a wider public. Since his death, over 1,000 new practitioners have been trained and accredited. Two authors of this book (David Zemach-Bersin and Mark Reese) were fortunate to be among the first Americans to study with Dr. Feldenkrais. They spent over ten years studying and working closely with him in both the United States and Europe. In 1983, they joined forces and began to collaborate on the development of **Relaxercise**,™ an exercise system designed to make the benefits of Feldenkrais's remarkable neuromuscular exercises available to *everyone* who would like to feel better.

This book is an introduction to both Relaxercise and the genius of Feldenkrais. It contains ten basic exercises to improve your health and well-being. Welcome to Relaxercise—we are sure you will enjoy the exercises and find them the easiest, most pleasant way to maintain a healthy, youthful, pain-free body.

This is the most sophisticated and effective method I have seen for the prevention and reversal of deterioration of function. . . . We're condemning millions of people to a deteriorated old age that's not necessary.

Margaret Mead, Ph.D., Anthropologist

The exercises are ingenuous and simple.

Yehudi Menuhin, Concert Violinist

Feldenkrais . . . represents a revolution in human health.

Albert Rosenfeld, *Smithsonian Magazine*

The system developed by Dr. Feldenkrais . . . has as much potential for understanding the mind/body relationship as Einstein's general theory of relativity had for physics.

Bernard Lake, M.D., Australia

He's not just pushing muscles around, but changing things in the brain itself.

Karl Pribram, M.D., Stanford University

Feldenkrais [has] had remarkable success in . . . a wide range of complaints ranging from the debilitating . . . to the merely nagging.

Science Digest

Dr. Moshe Feldenkrais's method will be of great benefit to all of humanity.

David Ben-Gurion, First Prime Minister of Israel

Feldenkrais has studied the body in movement with a precision that I have found nowhere else. He perfected hundreds of exercises of exceptional value.

Peter Brook, Film and Stage Director

HOW RELAXERCISE WORKS

Scientific discoveries have demonstrated that your *brain and nervous system* are the command and control center for your entire body. Relaxercise works to revitalize and improve your body by **enhancing the communication** between your brain and the rest of your body. By using the powerful connection between your brain and body, Relaxercise can bring about extraordinary physical changes and improvements with astounding efficiency and speed.

When we were small children, we learned how to sit up, roll over, crawl, stand, walk, and run. These accomplishments were achieved through an important natural process of trial and error. To learn how to walk, we first had to learn to stand up, maintain our balance, and take a single step. Only after falling down and getting up, over and over again, were we finally able to take many steps, one after another, without losing our balance and falling down.

Scientists call this process **sensory motor learning**. "Sensory motor," because it involves the use of our senses—sight, hearing, balance, and touch—in conjunction with movement. And "learning," because as a result, we *learn* how to do something new.

Sensory motor learning is how all physical learning takes place. It occurs through an information feedback process between your senses, muscles, and brain. As your body moves, your senses of touch, balance, and sight send your brain information about your body's position and muscular activity. Your brain responds by modifying the outgoing messages to your muscles. As the information is fed back and forth, the counterproductive and unnecessary muscular effort in your body is detected and "weeded out." Bit by bit, your movement becomes more refined and efficient. Information is exchanged between the brain and the senses until a successful, coordinated pattern of action is formed. Miraculously, the entire process takes place with virtually *no* conscious effort.

Remember when you learned to ride a bicycle? In the beginning, simply getting on the bike was a challenge. Although you held on very tight and made an enormous effort to keep your balance, you fell down many times. But with trial and error, you learned how to balance even while pedaling fast and turning corners. As your brain gradually reduced more and more of your body's unnecessary muscular effort, successful neuromuscular patterns were formed, and your bike-riding skills improved. Ultimately, you could keep your balance, pedal, watch the road, daydream, whistle a tune, and even take your hands off the handle bars, all at the same time.

Relaxercise is the first exercise system to improve your body by stimulating and using your brain's natural process of sensory motor learning.

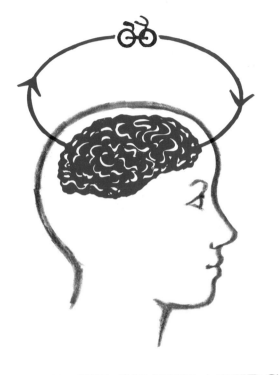

OUTGOING:
Improved regulation of
your postural orientation
and muscular activity

INCOMING:
New sensory information
about your posture and
muscular activity.

THE SECRET OF RELAXERCISE

In order to take advantage of your body's extraordinary ability to improve itself through sensory motor learning, you must give your brain an opportunity to detect and reduce the unnecessary, counterproductive muscular effort in your body. Research in neurophysiology has shown that when we exert a lot of *muscular effort, it is impossible for our brain to make the sensory distinctions needed to improve our neuromuscular organization.* This is why conventional exercise, with its reliance on muscular effort, force, and speed, actually restricts your brain's ability to work on your body's behalf. When we use *minimal* muscular effort, our brain is free to make important sensory distinctions.

For example: If you hold a heavy object, you have to exert a considerable amount of muscular effort. If a fly lands on top of the heavy object as you're holding it, you cannot feel the very slight increase in weight. This is because the muscular effort in your body is making it impossible for your brain to perceive the small change or difference in weight. But if you hold something that is very light, like a feather, you do not need to exert a lot of muscular effort. If a fly lands on the feather, you can easily feel the increase in weight because your brain is free to sense even the slightest difference or change.

Relaxercise exercises apply the powerful neurological rule: **less muscular effort produces more sensory motor learning, and physical improvement.**

The ten Relaxercise exercises in this book involve slow, easy movements that activate your brain's movement centers and generate a flow of valuable information between your brain and your muscles. Automatically, as if by magic, tension, strain, fatigue, and discomfort will disappear as your neuro-muscular system reprograms itself for better health.

THE BENEFITS OF RELAXERCISE

GOOD-BYE ACHES AND PAINS

Most aches and pains are due to a combination of muscular tension, strain, and poor posture. Relaxercise has an immediate soothing effect, relaxing your tired muscles, relieving strain and improving your posture. Your aches and pains can disappear very quickly—even chronic pains that may have been troubling you for a very long time. The exercises in this book will also help you to prevent their recurrence.

RELIEVE MUSCULAR TENSION

Muscular tension develops when you form an unconscious habit of using more muscular effort than you need to, or when your muscles remain contracted even when not in use. Sometimes the cause of muscular tension is emotional, and other times it's physical. But whatever the cause, tension habits frequently become chronic, and cause muscular pain, restricted movement, fatigue, and depression. Relaxercise will give you techniques to relieve muscular tension and to help you relax your muscles whenever you want.

INCREASE YOUR FLEXIBILITY

Your body needs to be flexible in order to maintain the health of your joints and muscles, and move with comfort and ease. As Relaxercise dissolves unhealthy neuromuscular habits of stiffness and tension, your flexibility will increase dramatically. When your body is more flexible, you will feel freer and healthier in ways you may not have felt in many years.

REDUCE YOUR STRESS LEVEL

As we all know, too much stress isn't good for you. It creates muscular tension and can cause jaw, chest, neck, shoulder, and back pain. Because the cause of stress is frequently beyond your control, your job is to reduce the level of muscular tension in your body and minimize its harmful effects. Relaxercise is an effective antidote to stress. It can provide quick relief and help prevent muscular tension from developing again.

DISCOVER DYNAMIC POSTURE

Your posture is extremely important. It affects your appearance, flexibility, freedom of movement, comfort, energy level, and future health. Postural habits are often considered very hard to change. But, with Relaxercise, your posture can improve quickly and easily. Relaxercise changes old postural habits by stimulating your nervous system's natural mechanisms for maintaining good posture. As your posture improves, you will begin to look and feel younger, you will experience less muscular tension, and your joints and muscles will be protected from harmful wear and tear.

Your **sitting posture** is important, too. Poor sitting posture is often responsible for the development of chronic levels of muscular tension and neck, shoulder, and back discomfort. If your occupation requires you to sit for more than four hours each day, your sitting posture should be one of your primary health concerns. In order to give special attention to improving sitting posture, seven of the exercises in this book can be done while seated. Relaxercise will directly improve your sitting posture and help combat the myriad aches and pains associated with long periods of sitting.

ENHANCE YOUR SPORTS PERFORMANCE

Relaxercise incorporates recent discoveries in neurophysiology and biomechanics to improve your neuromuscular organization. You may combine Relaxercise with all other forms of exercise. Warm up or cool down with Relaxercise or use Relaxercise to improve specific athletic skills. You will experience greater flexibility and efficiency of movement, more power and speed, improved accuracy and coordination in all your athletic activities.

REFRESH & REVITALIZE!

Relaxercise can increase your natural vitality and rejuvenate your body. Muscular tension, pain, and inefficient posture can drain your energy, leaving you tired and depleted. Relaxercise effectively relieves muscular tension, eliminates pain, and improves your posture. Try Relaxercise when you are feeling worn out and need an energy boost.

QUICK RECOVERY

After an injury or strain, Relaxercise can speed the healing process by relaxing your muscles, reducing inflammation, and stimulating your circulation. Sometimes an injury causes discomfort that lingers for months or even years. Often this is because we unconsciously develop compensatory posture and movement habits in order to avoid irritation of the injured area. These self-protective habits can persist long after the pain has gone and may cause chronic misalignment and muscular discomfort. Relaxercise helps you recover fully by dissolving old postural and movement habits that are no longer necessary and by reconditioning your body with healthier neuromuscular patterns.

MINIMIZE THE EFFECTS OF AGING

It is often assumed that poor posture, stiffness, and pain are unavoidable aspects of getting older. But this is *not* so! Many of the physical discomforts we accept as time goes by can be easily avoided. Relaxercise exercises improve your flexibility, posture, and freedom of movement, at *any* age.

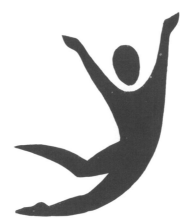

Relaxercise to the Rescue

Your body will benefit from *all* the Relaxercise exercises. This chart is intended to help you find those that may have special value for you.

If You Have:	Try Exercise Number:							
LOW BACK PAIN	1	2	3	5	6	7		
SHOULDER PAIN	1	4	6	7				
NECK ACHE	1	3	4	6	7	9		
HIP JOINT PAIN	1	2	3	5	8			
POOR POSTURE	1	2	3	4	5	6	8	10
FOOT/ANKLE PAIN	1	5	8					
HEADACHE	1	3	4	7	9	10		
CHRONIC TENSION	4	7	9					
SCOLIOSIS	1	2	3	4	5	6	7	
KNEE INJURY	1	5	8					
WHIPLASH INJURY	1	3	4	6	7	9		
JAW TENSION	4	7	9	10				
SCIATICA	1	3	4	5	7	8		
SHORTNESS OF BREATH	1	2	3	4	7	9		
EYESTRAIN	1	7	9	10				
SITTING DISCOMFORT	1	2	3	4	5	6	10	
FATIGUE	1	2	4	5	7			
MUSCLE STIFFNESS	1	2	4	5	6	7	9	

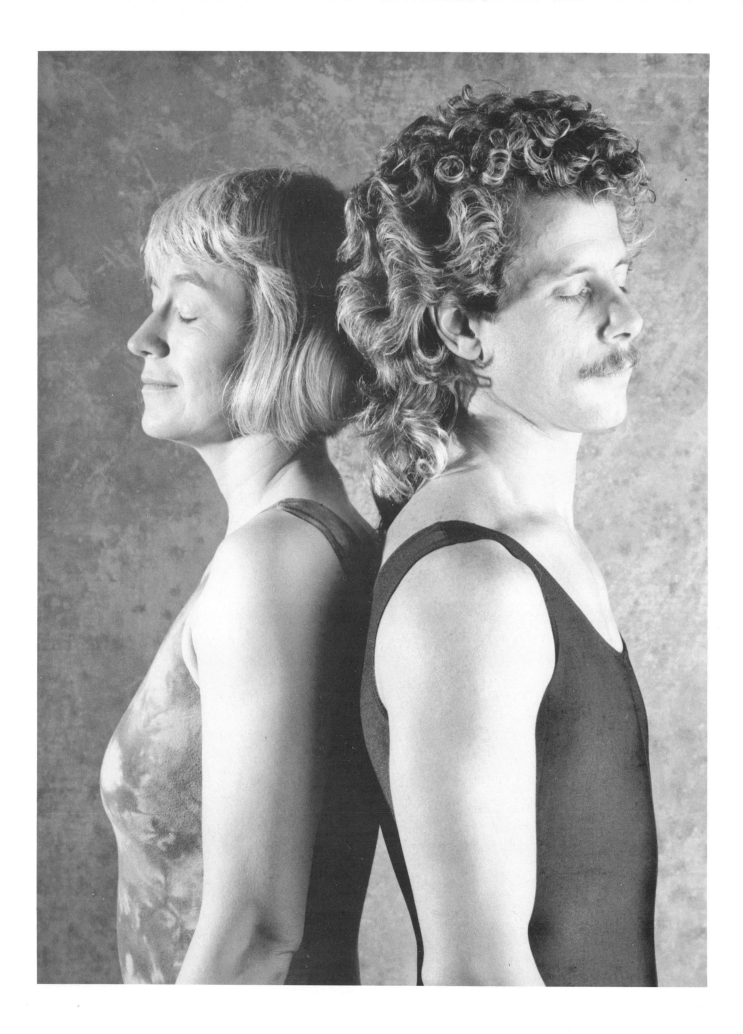

BEFORE YOU BEGIN

- You can do Relaxercise almost anywhere, and you can wear any sort of clothing.

- Start with any one of the ten exercises in this book. It is **not** necessary to do the exercises in the order in which they are presented. To begin, simply read the titles and choose an exercise you think might be especially useful for you.

- Each exercise is designed to take from fifteen to thirty minutes, depending on your individual style and pace. When you become familiar with an exercise, you can gain its benefits after doing the exercise for only a few minutes.

- In the beginning, repeat each exercise two or three times before moving on to a new one.

- Your body will improve quickly if the exercises are done on a regular basis. In the beginning, try to do one every day or every other day. Consistent use of Relaxercise initiates a process of steady improvement.

- Use a broad selection of the exercises in this book so your entire body can benefit from Relaxercise.

- Do not do more than two or three exercises per day. Your brain and body need adequate time between exercises to integrate the improvements.

- With Relaxercise it is **how** you do the movements that really counts, not how many times you repeat them. We suggest that you repeat each movement **at least** four to eight times. However, if you find some of the movements particularly beneficial, feel free to repeat them as many times as you like—even twenty to thirty times.

- Whenever possible, avoid stressful activities immediately after doing a Relaxercise exercise. This will help you to maintain the benefits of the exercise.

- Once you are familiar with the exercises, you may adapt them to custom fit your needs. If you wish, you may shorten the exercises by repeating each movement two or three times instead of the standard four to eight times. You may abbreviate, expand, or abridge the exercises freely, as long as you keep the Relaxercise **"Keys for Success"** in mind.

STARTING POSITIONS

Relaxercise exercises can be done either while seated, or lying down.

Sitting exercises: If your shoes are uncomfortable, or if you are wearing high heels, please remove them. Choose a chair with a hard or firmly cushioned seat. The seat should be low enough to allow your feet to rest flat on the floor, comfortably. If the seat is too high, you can raise the floor level under each foot by resting your feet on two books of equal height.

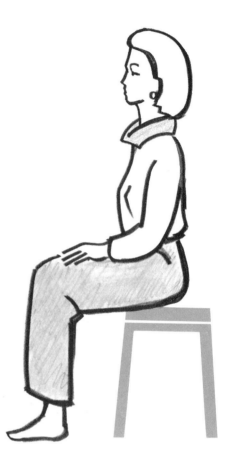

Floor exercises: Please remove your shoes. Choose a firmly cushioned surface, such as an exercise mat or rug. If due to an injury or disability, you are unable to lie on the floor comfortably, you may do Relaxercise while lying in bed.

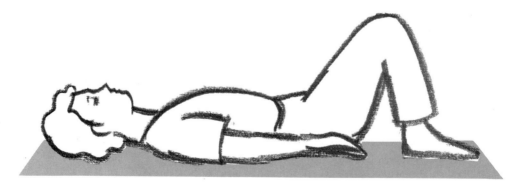

THE RELAXERCISE KEYS FOR SUCCESS

To make the benefits of Relaxercise yours, use the "Keys for Success." These guidelines are **very** important. They will ensure that each exercise is communicated effectively to your brain and body. Read the keys carefully before you begin.

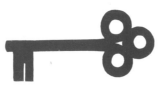

Make Each Movement Easy

As you do each movement, use as **little** muscular effort as possible. Do not strain or stretch your body. Make each movement **small, comfortable and easy.**

Go Slowly

Do each movement **slowly**—so you can pay attention to what you feel and become aware of unnecessary muscular effort in your body.

Relax as Much as You Can

As you do each movement, try to let go of tension and relax. This is an important aspect of Relaxercise.

Rest Briefly After Each Movement

Do not repeat the movements quickly, one after another. Rest for a few moments between each movement. This will give your brain the time it needs to absorb new and useful sensory motor information.

IN CASE OF DISCOMFORT OR LIMITATION

You should **never** experience discomfort or pain while doing a Relaxercise exercise. Pain indicates physical irritation. If you begin to experience **any** physical discomfort at all, respond by making each movement extra small, extra slight, and extra easy—or just **imagine** doing the movements without actually moving.

Discomfort **after** an exercise may indicate that you used too much muscular effort while doing the movements. Take a minute to review the Relaxercise "Keys for Success" and next time you do an exercise, don't do "too much." If you stay well within the limits of your body's natural comfort zone, each Relaxercise exercise will be an enjoyable and beneficial experience.

Relaxercise is an unusually effective and safe form of exercise. The exercises in this book are suitable for everyone, and may be used at any time, including during pregnancy and while recovering from an injury.

Occasionally, pain, injury, or physical limitation may interfere with your ability to do an exercise. In almost all cases, you can still benefit from the exercise by making each movement extremely small and slow. The exercises in this book are ideal for helping your body to heal and repair itself. As you do an exercise, make each movement very slight. Make sure that each movement feels completely comfortable and easy. You can also experiment with doing the movements in your imagination. This is a technique called visualization, and it can be very useful.

Research has shown that your brain's electrical activity is essentially the same when you imagine doing a movement as when you physically do it. When you imagine or **visualize** moving, your brain sends messages to your muscles identical to the ones it sends when you actually move your body. The only difference is that when you visualize moving, the messages are not intense enough to make your muscles fully contract. Visualization is a powerful tool and can be as effective and beneficial as physically doing the movements.

To visualize the movements of an exercise, just close your eyes and imagine that you are doing the movements—**without** actually moving your body.

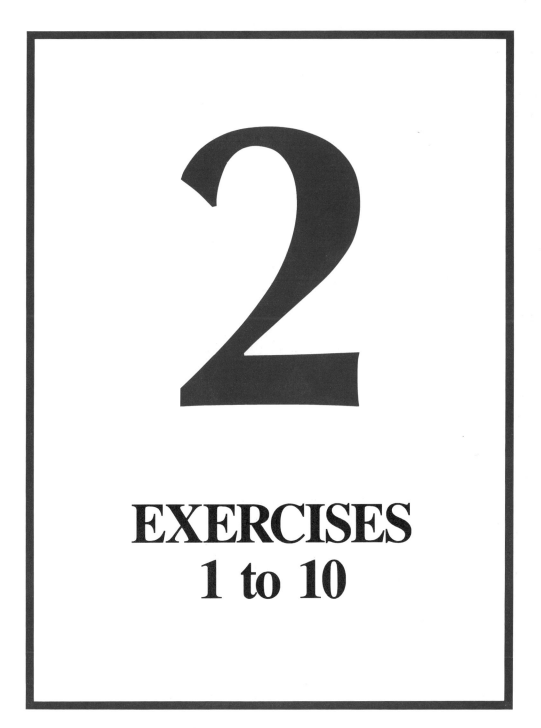

2

EXERCISES
1 to 10

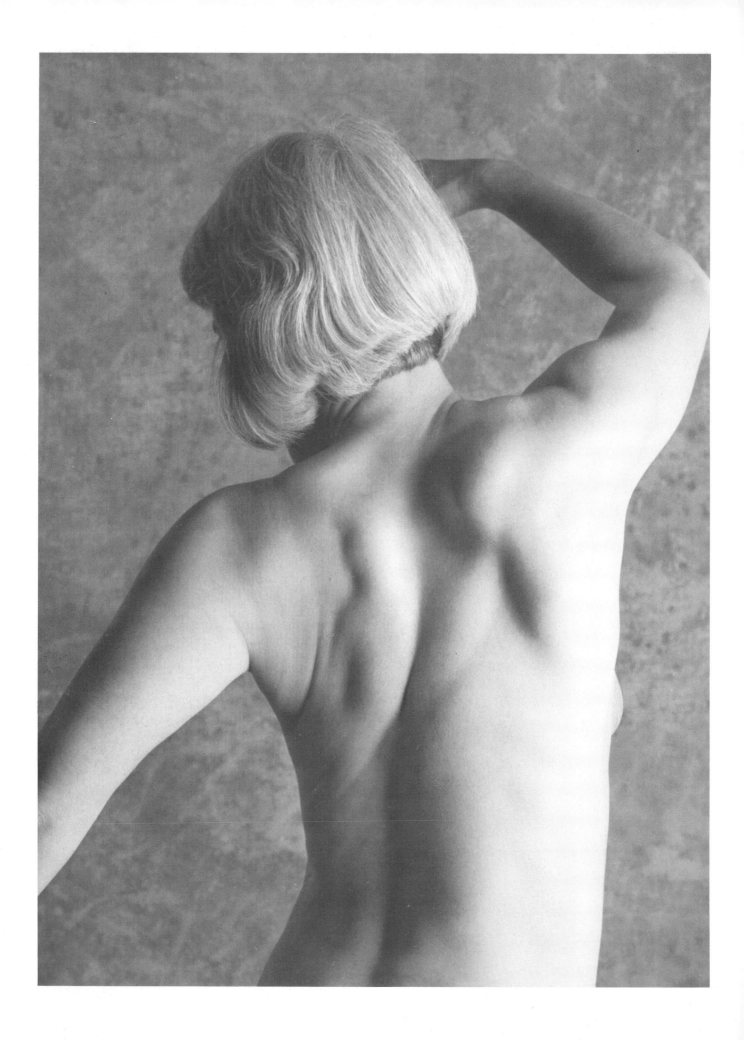

1 EASY FLEXIBILITY

Sandra K., a thirty-two-year-old executive producer for a West Coast television station, was concerned about her decreasing flexibility. Though young and naturally athletic, two automobile accidents and a high-stress job left her with the flexibility of someone twice her age. By using "Easy Flexibility," Sandra increased the flexibility of her neck, chest, and spine by more than 80 percent in only a few days. By doing Relaxercise at home and during breaks at work, she soon regained her flexibility and ease of movement.

Turning is a vital element in almost every movement we make. Literally thousands of times each day, we turn our body left and right. Activities such as walking or running require us to turn with every step. Even the simplest actions, like reaching for a pen or putting on our shoes, involve numerous small turning movements.

It is the marvelous engineering of your spine that makes turning possible. Your spine is composed of thirty-three vertebrae. In fact, the word *vertebra* comes from the Latin word *vertere*, which means "to turn." When you turn, each vertebra rotates only a few degrees. But the combined rotation of all your vertebrae allows you to turn from 90 to 180 degrees, far enough to see all the way behind yourself.

For nearly all of us, our ability to turn freely and easily becomes restricted by the time we reach adulthood. You may experience stiffness and discomfort when you are engaged in a particular activity, like turning to look over your shoulder while driving. Or you may simply notice that you no longer have the flexibility and freedom of movement you used to enjoy. When your freedom to turn becomes restricted, your posture suffers, you feel less energetic, and you are more vulnerable to neck, shoulder, and back problems.

"Easy Flexibility" will dramatically increase your comfort while turning and will help restore your natural flexibility. It will improve your posture and leave you feeling more energetic.

EASY FLEXIBILITY

You will need a hard or firmly cushioned chair or seat.

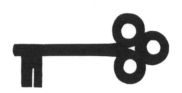

Use the Relaxercise Keys

- **Go slowly.**

- **Make each movement small and easy.**

- **Relax as much as you can.**

- **Rest briefly after each movement.**

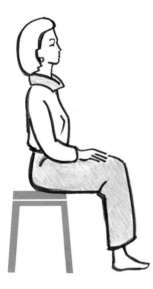

STARTING POSITION
Sit on the forward part of your chair or seat and rest your hands on your thighs.
Rest your feet flat on the floor, shoulder width apart, directly below your knees.

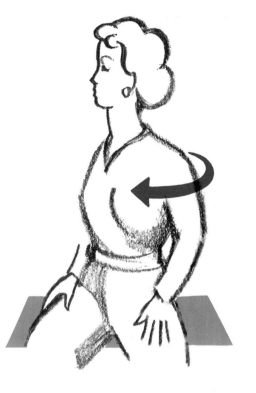

Slowly turn your upper body, as if to look to the right a little. Then return to facing forward and relax.

- Make each movement small, comfortable, and easy.
- Keep your feet flat on the floor.
- Make a mental note of exactly how far to the right you can see, without feeling *any* strain. Later this will be a point of reference when you measure the improvement in your flexibility.

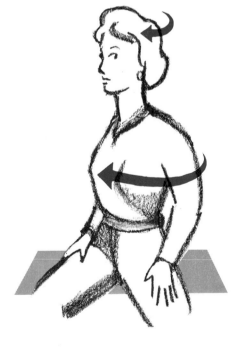

Focus your eyes on an object or spot straight ahead. Keep your eyes still, looking straight ahead, while slowly turning your head and upper body to the right. Then return to facing forward and relax.

- Don't use force; don't stretch or strain.
- To make the movement easier, exhale as you turn.
- Relax your neck, shoulders, chest, and legs.
- Notice that your upper body doesn't turn as far to the right, because your eyes are not moving.

pause to rest after each movement

3 Once again, slowly turn your *entire* upper body to the right, including your eyes.

- Turn your head, eyes, shoulders, and chest, gently.
- Can you see a little farther to the right?

4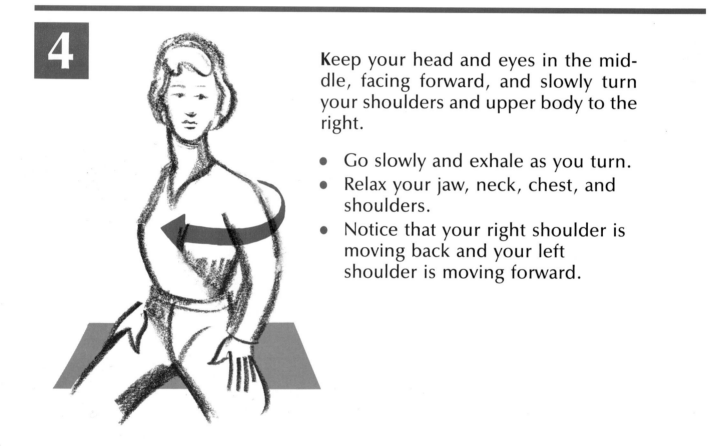

Keep your head and eyes in the middle, facing forward, and slowly turn your shoulders and upper body to the right.

- Go slowly and exhale as you turn.
- Relax your jaw, neck, chest, and shoulders.
- Notice that your right shoulder is moving back and your left shoulder is moving forward.

5 Again, slowly turn your entire upper body to the right, including your head and eyes. Then return to the starting position and relax.

- Notice how turning to the right is becoming easier and more comfortable!

your flexibility will increase automatically

And now, rest.

- Feel the difference between your left and right shoulder.
- Feel how your left side is relaxing!

6

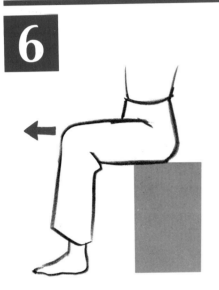

Keep your foot still and flat on the floor, but move your left knee forward very slightly.

- This is a very small movement.
- Relax your left leg and foot as much as possible.
- Notice that your lower back, head, and shoulders are turning slightly to the right.

7

Simultaneously, move your left knee forward slowly, while turning your entire upper body to the right.

- Notice that you get a little taller as you turn.
- Exhale as you turn so your chest can be more flexible.
- As you turn, feel how your pelvis moves a little.
- Notice that moving your left knee forward improves your ability to turn.

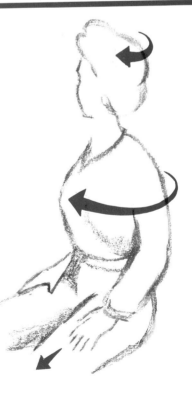

relax your neck, back, stomach and legs

And now, rest.

- Notice that your left shoulder and the left side of your neck and lower back are more relaxed.
- Feel the difference!

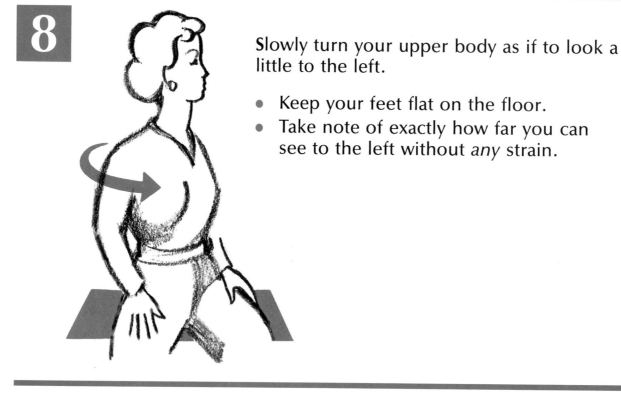

8

Slowly turn your upper body as if to look a little to the left.

- Keep your feet flat on the floor.
- Take note of exactly how far you can see to the left without *any* strain.

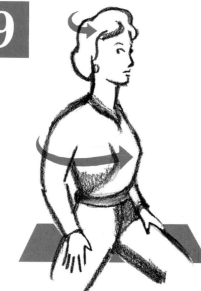

9

Focus your eyes on an object or spot straight ahead. Keep your eyes in the middle, facing forward, while slowly turning your head and upper body to the left.

- Relax your face, neck, shoulders, and legs.
- Notice that your upper body does not turn as far as before, because your eyes are staying still.

make each movement slow and easy

go slowly so your muscles can relax

10 Again, turn your upper body, including your eyes, to the left.

- Turn comfortably, without any strain.
- Can you see a little farther to the left than before?

---

11 Keep your head and eyes in the middle, facing forward, while slowly turning your shoulders and upper body to the left.

- Relax your face, neck, shoulders, and stomach as much as you can.
- Feel how your left shoulder moves back and your right shoulder moves forward.

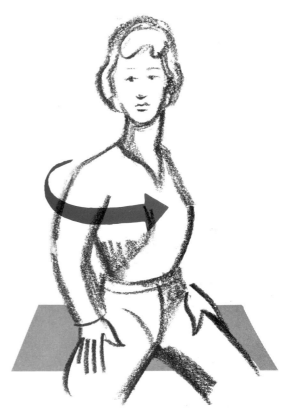

---

12 Again, turn your upper body, including your head and eyes, to the left.

- Feel how much easier this movement has become!
- Notice that as you turn left, your right knee naturally moves forward a little.

exhale as you do each movement

13 Keep your foot flat on the floor, and move your right knee forward very slightly.

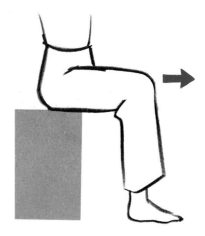

- After each movement, let your knee return to the starting position and rest.
- Don't push with your right leg or foot.
- Notice that your right buttock and hip move forward slightly.
- Relax your right leg completely.
- Notice that your lower back, head, and shoulders turn slightly to the left.

14

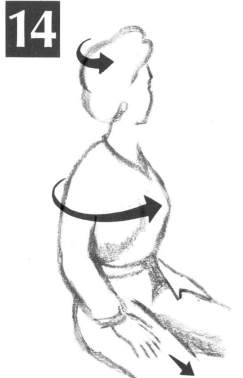

Move your right knee forward slightly, while turning your upper body to the left.

- Notice that your body gets a little taller as you turn.
- Relax your neck, shoulders, arms, back, and legs.
- Feel the slight movement of your pelvis.
- Notice how much farther to the left you are turning!

And now, rest.

- Feel how relaxed your right side is!

feel the difference! and then continue . . .

15 Move your left knee forward very slightly, while slowly turning your entire upper body to the right. Then return—go through the starting position—and move your right knee forward, while slowly turning your entire upper body to the left.

- Make the movement smooth and continuous.
- Let your hands slide on your thighs as you turn from side to side.
- Relax your legs as much as possible.

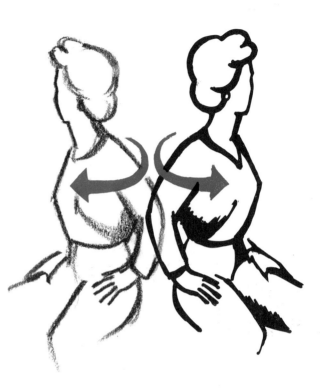

16

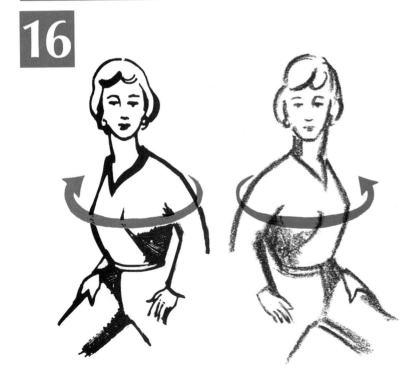

Keep your head and eyes still, facing forward, and continue turning the rest of your upper body to the right a little—and to the left a little.

- Relax your face, neck, and shoulders.
- Keep your feet flat on the floor.
- Breathe freely.

stop and rest whenever you like

use as little effort as possible

17 Turn your entire upper body to the right and then to the left.

- As you turn to the right, notice that your left shoulder moves forward and your right shoulder moves back.
- As you turn to the left, notice that your right shoulder moves forward and your left shoulder moves back.
- Feel how much your flexibility has increased!

---

18 Alternately, turn your upper body and pelvis to the right, while turning your head and eyes to the left—and slowly turn your upper body and pelvis to the left, while turning your head and eyes to the right.

- Go slowly so the movement is smooth and easy.
- Don't stretch or strain. Your flexibility will increase automatically.
- Relax your jaw, neck, shoulders, and legs as much as you can.
- Breathe freely.

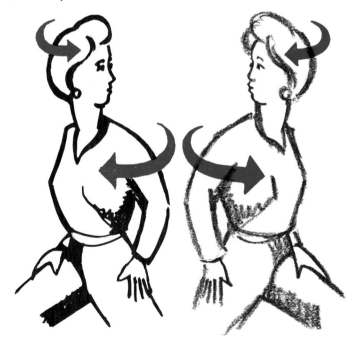

alternate slowly 4 to 8 times

let your body move freely

19

Now, measure your improvement: Move your left knee forward while turning your entire upper body to the right as far as you can, without any strain. Then move your right knee forward while turning your entire upper body to the left as far as you can, without any strain.

- Notice how easily you are turning and how much farther to the right and left you can see!
- Feel how much your flexibility has increased without any stretching or force!

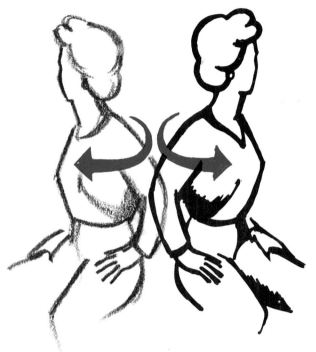

And now, rest.

Feel how comfortably you are sitting! Your weight is now balanced evenly on your pelvic sitting bones and your lower back is slightly arched. You may feel and look a little taller. This is because your muscles are relaxed and your posture is more upright. Sit this way whenever possible. Your back will strengthen, you will avoid aches and pains, and you will feel more energetic!

You have completed **"Easy Flexibility."** When you stand up and walk around, notice how light and relaxed your body feels and how comfortably you are moving.

Enjoy the improvement!

YOUR BACK

Back pain is a modern problem of epidemic proportions. It is estimated that 80 percent of us suffer severe back pain at some time in our lives. Each year an estimated 19 million Americans consult physicians on account of their back problems, and almost 100 million workdays are lost each year due to back trouble.

Your spine consists of twenty-four separate vertebrae and nine vertebrae that are fused together at the base of the spine. Between the separate vertebrae are pads (discs) of tough connective tissue which act as shock-absorbing cushions. Your spine is supported and stabilized by your ribs, pelvis, muscles, and ligaments.

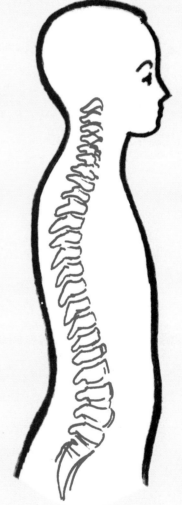

Your spine:

1. Supports the weight of your upper body.
2. Distributes the weight of your upper body to your legs via your pelvis.
3. Makes your back flexible.
4. Protects your spinal cord and nerves.
5. Connects your head, chest, and pelvis.

The structural health of your spine is maintained by four natural curves. The curves of your lower back and neck are concave, and the curves of your upper back and tailbone are convex. The long S-shaped curve of your spine gives your back flexibility and maximizes its strength and capacity to absorb compression.

Medical experts agree that our sedentary life-styles and occupations are the most common causes of back pain today. Many of us sit relatively still for eight to fifteen hours every day. Sitting increases the pressure on your spine and discs by as much as 50 percent, and when you sit for long periods of time, your back generally becomes rounded. This diminishes the natural curves of your spine and increases the amount of mechanical and muscular stress in your back. When your back is rounded, your discs are more compressed, your back muscles are overstretched, and your posture invariably suffers. For sitting posture solutions, see The Art of Dynamic Sitting, page 137.

When the arch of your lower back is severely diminished for a long period of time, the pressure on one of your discs can become so extreme that it may herniate or rupture. A ruptured disc can cause irritation of the sciatic nerve, which can lead to one of the most painful and debilitating types of back problems, commonly called *"sciatica."*

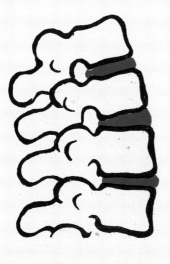 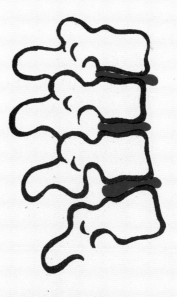

**Healthy alignment
of lower back**

**Unhealthy alignment
of lower back**

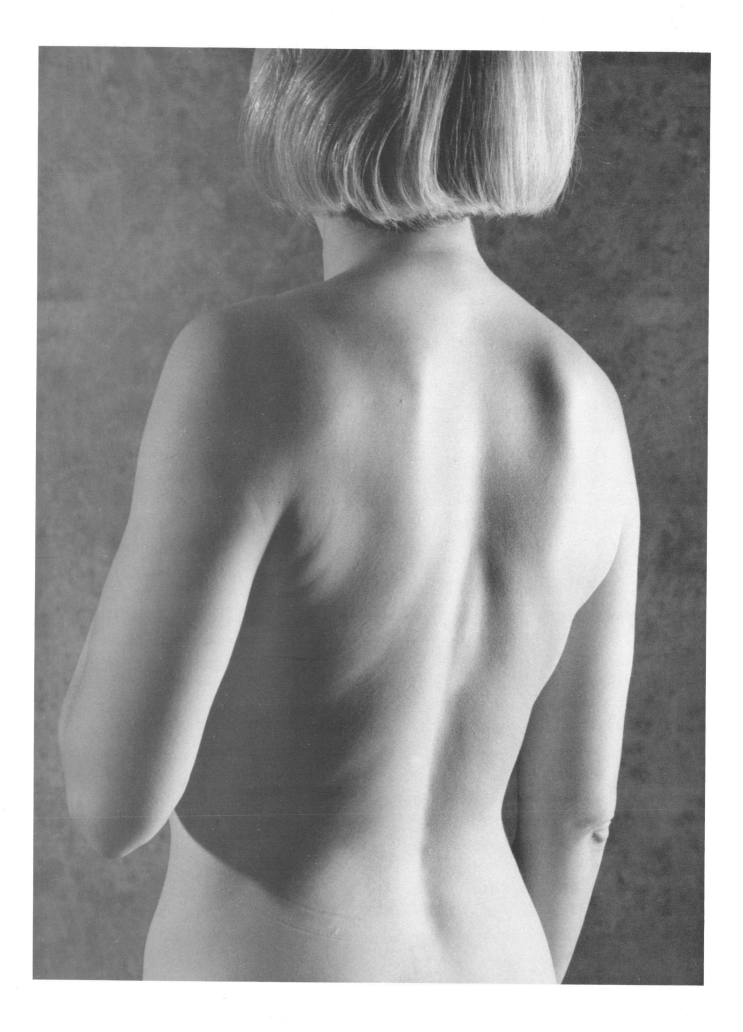

2 LOW BACK COMFORT

Carl S., a forty-four-year-old high school teacher, felt himself to be in a perpetual state of tension and pain. Carl was forced to take a medical leave of absence. A devoted and ambitious teacher, Carl felt he was being defeated by his own body. But with Relaxercise, Carl found complete relief. He soon returned to work and was successfully able to prevent recurrence of the back tension and pain he had become so accustomed to.

Back care is something we should **all** know about. Nearly one of every two Americans has experienced serious back problems, and over 250,000 people have back surgery each year. These figures could be much lower if we had a basic understanding of how our back works, what its limitations are, and how to protect our back from becoming strained and weakened.

Most back problems develop gradually, as the result of poor posture and excessive muscular tension and strain. Because our backs are naturally very strong, it can take many years of stress and abuse before we begin to feel weakness or discomfort.

Each back problem is unique, but there are common symptoms: chronic muscular tension, restricted flexibility, poor postural organization, and pain. Back pain can affect your emotional disposition, your ability to function and can trigger neck, shoulder, and chest pain as well.

"Low Back Comfort" is designed to reduce muscular tension in your back and improve the balance of muscular tonus between your abdomen and lower back. When your lower back is relaxed and comfortable, your spine will support your body's weight more efficiently, and you will be less vulnerable to back problems.

LOW BACK COMFORT

You will need an exercise mat or rug.

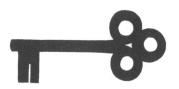

Use the Relaxercise Keys

- **Go slowly.**

- **Make each movement small and easy.**

- **Relax as much as you can.**

- **Rest briefly after each movement.**

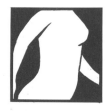

NOTE: This exercise consists of four sets of movements. Each set has its own **SPECIAL** starting position.

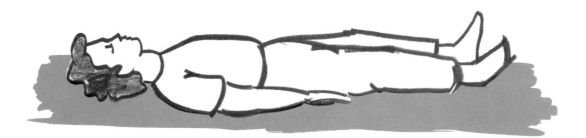

BEFORE YOU BEGIN:

Lie on your back and stretch out your legs.
Rest your arms by your sides.
For a minute or two, feel **how** your back is
lying on the floor.

- Feel how your legs are resting on the floor. Does one leg feel slightly longer or more relaxed than the other?
- Notice that some parts of your lower back are touching the floor and other parts are not.
- Feel how your spine is resting on the floor. Notice that some of your vertebrae are touching the floor more clearly than others.
- Feel how your shoulder blades are lying on the floor. Is one shoulder blade lying in closer contact with the floor than the other?
- Feel how your arms are resting on the floor. Are your hands touching the floor in the same way, or differently?
- Feel the way your head is resting on the floor. Does it feel a little closer to the right shoulder or left shoulder, or is it exactly in the middle?

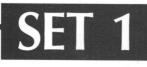

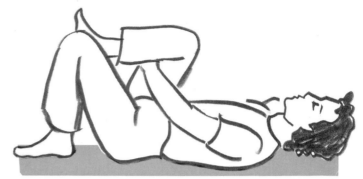

STARTING POSITION

Bend your knees. Place your feet flat on the floor, shoulder width apart, directly below your knees. Lift your right foot and bring your right knee toward your upper body. Hold your right leg by putting your left hand (including the thumb) behind your right knee.

Put your right hand behind your head and rest your elbow on the floor.

As you do movements A, B, and C:

- Go slowly.
- Make each movement small and easy. You don't need to touch your knee.
- Between each movement, return to the starting position and let your head and elbow return to the floor.
- Exhale as you do each movement, to make it easier.
- When you lift your head, notice how your right elbow moves forward and your forearm moves closer to your cheek.
- Support your head with your right hand.
- Relax your neck, arms, chest, stomach, and both legs.
- Notice which parts of your back move closer to the floor as you bend.
- As you do each movement, notice that your chest flattens and your back rounds.
- Use as little effort as possible, and you will improve quickly.

repeat each movement 4 to 8 times

and

pause to rest after each movement

A Simultaneously, lift your head with your right hand and slowly guide your right elbow toward your right knee, while your left hand slowly guides your right knee toward your right elbow.

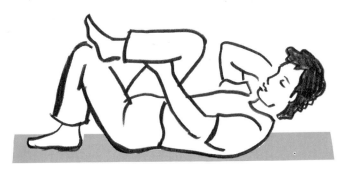

B Simultaneously, lift your head with your right hand and slowly guide your chin toward your right knee, while your left hand slowly guides your right knee toward your chin.

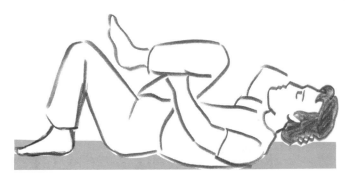

C Simultaneously, lift your head with your right hand, and slowly guide your forehead toward your right knee, while your left hand slowly guides your right knee toward your forehead.

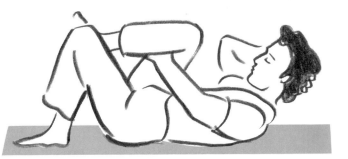

When you have finished A, B, and C, stretch out your legs, and relax. Notice that the right side of your back is resting closer to the floor. Feel how your entire right side is more relaxed than the left.

feel the difference! and then continue . . .

SET 2

STARTING POSITION

Bend your knees. Place your feet flat on the floor, shoulder width apart, directly under your knees. Lift your left foot and bring your left knee toward your upper body. Hold your left leg by putting your right hand (including the thumb) behind your left knee.
Put your left hand behind your head and let your elbow rest on the floor.

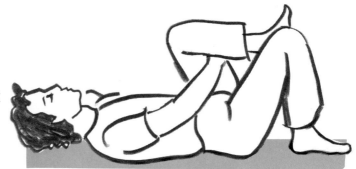

As you do movements A, B, and C:

- Go slowly.
- Between each movement, return to starting position and rest briefly.
- Make each movement slight, small, and easy.
- Use as little muscular effort as possible.
- Let your head and elbow return to the floor and pause to rest.
- Exhale as you do each movement, to make it easier.
- When you lift your head, notice that your left elbow moves forward and your forearm moves closer to your cheek.
- Support your head with your left hand.
- Relax your neck, arms, chest, stomach, and legs.
- Your left leg can relax and be passive.
- Notice which parts of your back move closer to the floor as you bend.
- As you do each movement, notice that your chest flattens and your back rounds.

repeat each movement 4 to 8 times

and

pause to rest after each movement

A Simultaneously, lift your head with your left hand and slowly guide your left elbow toward your left knee, while your right hand slowly guides your left knee toward your left elbow.

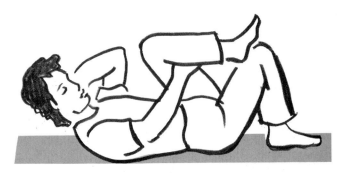

B Simultaneously, lift your head with your left hand and slowly guide your chin toward your left knee, while your right hand slowly guides your left knee toward your chin.

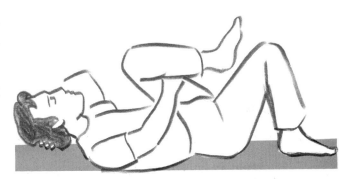

C Simultaneously, lift your head with your left hand and slowly guide your forehead toward your left knee, while your right hand slowly guides your left knee toward your fore-head.

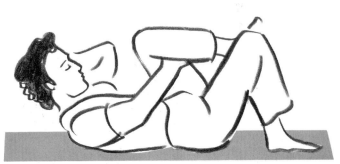

 When you have finished A, B, and C, stretch out your legs and relax. Notice that the left side of your back is resting closer to the floor. Feel how your entire left side is more relaxed.

feel the difference! and then continue . . .

STARTING POSITION

Bend your knees. Place your feet flat on the floor, shoulder width apart, directly under your knees. Lift your right foot and bring your right knee toward your upper body. Hold your right leg by putting your right hand (including the thumb) behind your right knee from the outside of your right leg.

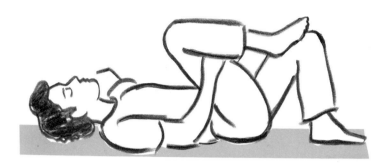

Put your left hand behind your head and let your elbow rest on the floor.

As you do movements A, B, and C:

- Note that this is a diagonal movement.
- Let your head and elbow return to the floor and rest between each movement.
- When you lift your head, notice how your left forearm moves closer to your cheek.
- Go slowly.
- Make each movement slight and small.
- Exhale as you do each movement, so that your back can bend more easily.
- Support your head with your left hand.
- Relax your neck, arms, chest, stomach, and legs.
- Your right leg can relax and be passive.
- As you bend, feel how certain parts of your back move closer to the floor.
- Relax so your chest can flatten.
- If you use minimal muscular effort, your muscles will lengthen naturally.

repeat each movement 4 to 8 times

and

pause to rest after each movement

A Simultaneously, lift your head with your left hand and slowly guide your left elbow toward your right knee, while your right hand slowly guides your right knee toward your left elbow.

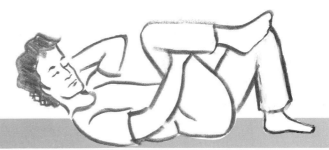

B Simultaneously, lift your head with your left hand and slowly guide your chin toward your right knee, while your right hand guides your right knee toward your chin.

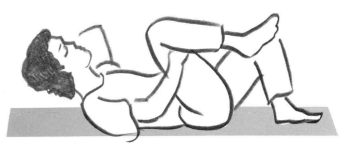

C Simultaneously, lift your head with your left hand and slowly guide your forehead toward your right knee, while your right hand slowly guides your right knee toward your forehead.

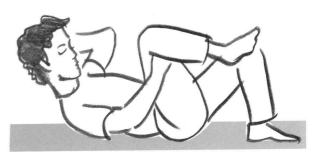

When you have finished A, B, and C, stretch out your legs and relax. Notice that more of your body is relaxing and is now in closer contact with the floor.

feel the difference! and then continue . . .

SET 4

STARTING POSITION

Bend your knees. Place your feet flat on the floor, shoulder width apart, directly under your knees. Lift your left foot and bring your left knee toward your upper body. Hold your left leg by putting your left hand (including the thumb) behind your left knee from the outside of your left leg.

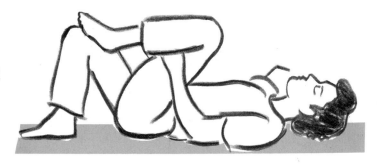

Put your right hand behind your head and let your elbow rest on the floor.

As you do movements A, B, and C:

- Notice that this is a diagonal movement.
- Let your head and elbow return to the floor and rest between each movement.
- When you lift your head, notice that your right forearm moves closer to the side of your face.
- Go slowly.
- Make each movement slight and small.
- Exhale as you do each movement.
- Support your head with your right hand.
- Relax your neck, arms, chest, stomach, and legs.
- Your right leg can relax and be passive.
- As you bend, feel how certain parts of your back move closer to the floor.
- If you use minimal muscular effort, your muscles will lengthen naturally.

repeat each movement 4 to 8 times

and

pause to rest after each movement

A **S**imultaneously, lift your head with your right hand and slowly guide your right elbow toward your left knee, while your left hand slowly guides your left knee toward your right elbow.

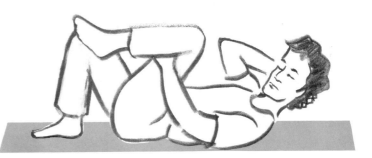

B **S**imultaneously, lift your head with your right hand and slowly guide your chin toward your left knee, while your left hand slowly guides your knee toward your chin.

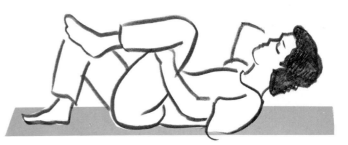

C **S**imultaneously, lift your head with your right hand and slowly guide your forehead toward your left knee, while your left hand slowly guides your left knee toward your forehead.

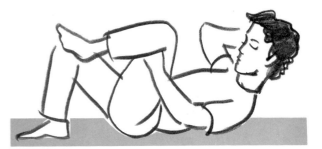

When you have finished movements A, B, and C, relax completely.

Notice that your entire body is resting closer to the floor. Your lower back may not have been this relaxed in years!
You have completed **"Low Back Comfort."** When you stand up and walk around, feel the improvement in your posture. Feel the freedom in your hip joints and the lightness as you walk.

Enjoy the improvement!

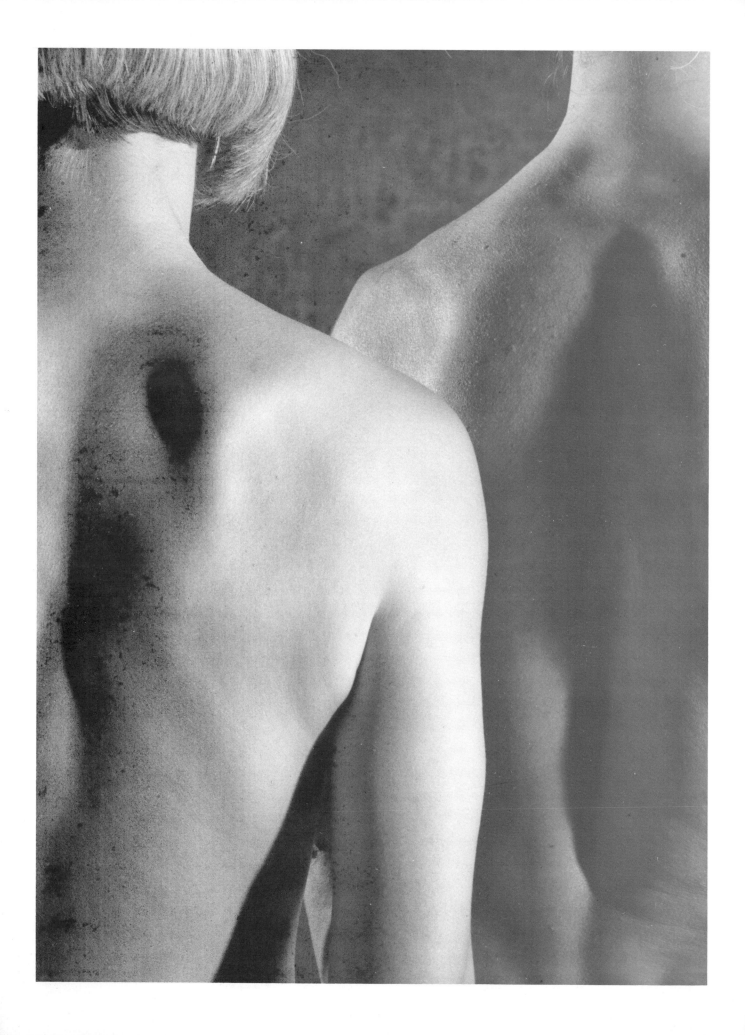

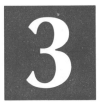

3 A HEALTHY SPINE

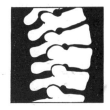

James N., a thirty-nine-year-old computer programmer, had slouched in his chair for nearly twenty years, twelve hours a day. Though he jogged five miles a day, he felt that his upper back was beginning to resemble the "Hunchback of Notre Dame," and his neck and shoulders ached severely every evening. Neither stretching exercises nor aspirin helped. Using Relaxercise, Jim was able to eliminate his neck and shoulder pain and improve his posture. By doing Relaxercise for a few minutes each day, he found that he could easily maintain a healthy, stress-free sitting posture while at work.

By the time we reach adulthood, our body's freedom of movement has often become significantly restricted. This is largely because most of our daily activities involve bending our spine in predominantly **one** direction—**forward**.

At home and at work, almost everything you do involves bending forward. Your spine's ability to move left, right, and especially backward is used less frequently. But bending freely in **all** directions is crucial to the health and comfort of your back.

Your spine is composed of two concave arches: the cervical arch of your neck and the lumbar arch of your lower back. These natural arches are essential to the flexibility of your spine and vital to its weight-bearing and shock-absorbing capabilities. It is a common misconception that a flat lower back and a straight neck comprise "good posture." These positions eliminate the important natural arches of your spine. Without healthy curves of the neck and lower back, your ligaments and discs become over-stressed, your muscles become overworked, your back gets tired more easily, and you are more vulnerable to strain and injury.

The many years of bending forward inevitably take their toll as we get older. The curves of our spine become weakened and are often completely lost. Bending backward becomes difficult and painful. This is why our posture tends to become more and more stooped in our later years.

To maintain the natural curves of your spine, you must keep your back flexible and be able to bend backward with comfort and ease. **"A Healthy Spine"** will help you to restore the health and flexibility of your spine, increase the freedom of movement in your neck and back, improve your posture, and help you bend more freely and easily in all directions.

A HEALTHY SPINE

You will need a hard or firmly cushioned chair or seat.

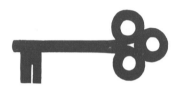

Use the Relaxercise Keys

- **Go slowly.**

- **Make each movement small and easy.**

- **Relax as much as you can.**

- **Rest briefly after each movement.**

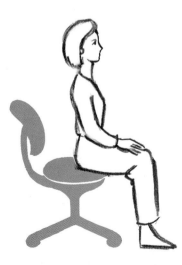

STARTING POSITION
Sit on the forward part of your chair or seat and rest your hands on your thighs.
Rest your feet flat on the floor, shoulder width apart, directly below your knees.

1

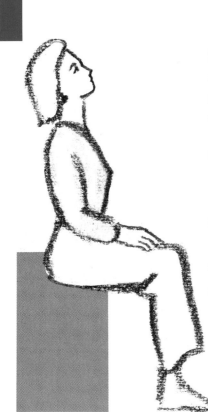

Slowly and comfortably raise your head and eyes as if to look up toward the ceiling. Then return to the starting position (facing forward) and relax.

- Don't stretch or strain your neck or back. Your flexibility will increase automatically.
- As you look up, let your back arch slightly.
- Exhale as you do each movement.
- As you look up, notice exactly how far above your eyes can see without feeling **any** strain. Later on, you can measure your improvement.

2

Simultaneously, raise your head and arch your back a little, while looking downward with your eyes.

- Go slowly. This movement will soon be easier and more comfortable.
- The movement of your head and neck is limited because your head and eyes are moving in opposite directions.
- Relax your eyes, neck, and shoulders.

rest in the starting position after each movement

3 Simultaneously, raise your head and eyes to look up toward the ceiling while arching your back.

- Is your back arching more easily?
- Can you see a little higher without *any* strain?

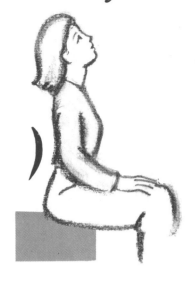

---

4 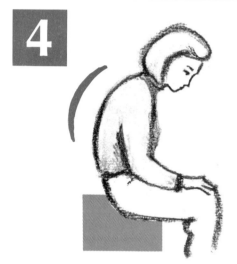 Very slowly lower your head as if to look down toward the floor. Then return to the starting position and relax.

- Make each movement small and easy.
- When you look down, let your back get round.
- Exhale as you do each movement.
- Relax your neck, chest, and shoulders.

---

5 Simultaneously, lower your head and round your back, while raising your eyes to look upward.

- Notice that the movement of your head and chest is limited because your head and eyes are moving in opposite directions.

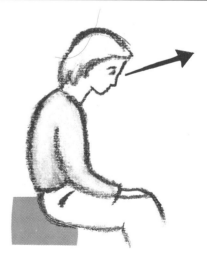

go slowly so your muscles can relax

6 Again, raise your head and eyes to look upward, while arching your back.

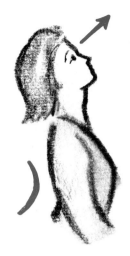

- Notice that your eyes can see a little farther upward without strain!
- Feel the middle and upper part of your back beginning to arch a little more.

7

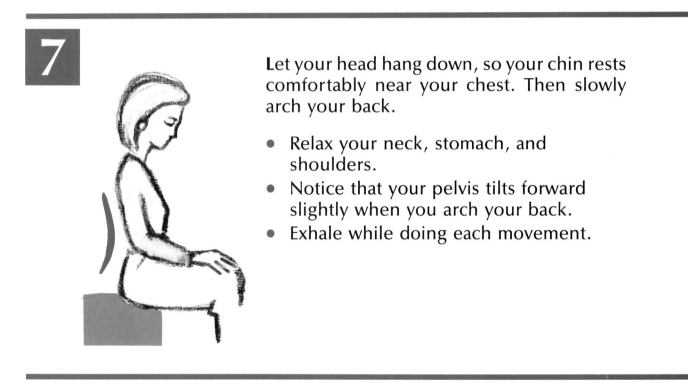

Let your head hang down, so your chin rests comfortably near your chest. Then slowly arch your back.

- Relax your neck, stomach, and shoulders.
- Notice that your pelvis tilts forward slightly when you arch your back.
- Exhale while doing each movement.

8 And once more, raise your head and eyes to look upward while arching your back.

- Feel your spine arching.
- Notice how far upward you can look now, without feeling any strain.

feel the difference! and then continue . . .

9

Slowly, lift your head and eyes to look upward, while arching your back. Then slowly lower your head and eyes and round your back.

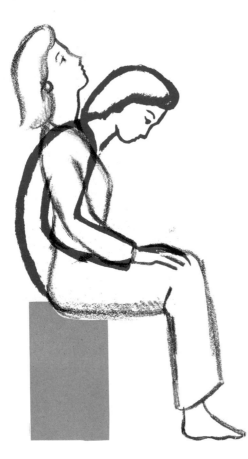

As you look **upward,** notice:

- Your shoulder blades move closer together.
- Your stomach relaxes and moves forward.
- Your pelvis tilts forward a little.
- Your chest lifts and moves forward.
- Your body gets a little taller.

As you look **downward,** notice:

- Your chest flattens.
- Your shoulders and back are rounded.
- Your pelvis tilts backward a little.
- Your body gets a little shorter.

stop to rest as often as you like

10

Turn your upper body comfortably to the right and stay there. Then alternately raise your head and eyes to look upward while arching your back, and then lower your head while rounding your back.

- Remain turned slightly to the right.
- Pause to rest when your head and eyes are lowered.
- To make the movement easier, lift your left hip slightly as you look up.
- Relax your neck, shoulders, and legs as much as possible.

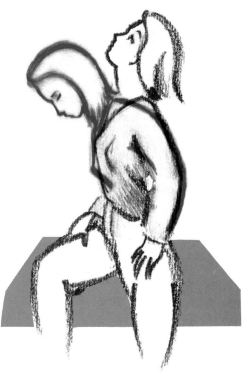

11

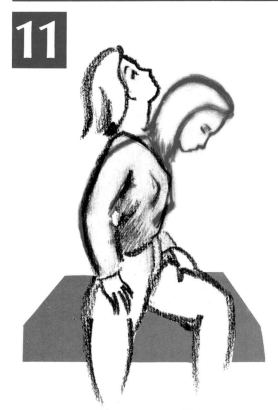

Turn your upper body comfortably to the left and stay there. Then alternately raise your head and eyes to look upward while arching your back, and then lower your head and eyes while rounding your back.

- Remain turned slightly to the left.
- As you look upward, lift your right hip slightly.
- Relax your neck, shoulders, and legs as much as you can.

make each movement slow, relaxed and easy

alternate 4 to 8 times

12

Slowly turn to the right, while arching your back and looking upward. Then, while lowering your head and rounding your back, bring your body back through the starting position and turn slowly to the left, while arching your back and looking upward. Lower your head and round your back as you bring your body through the starting position again and repeat the movement.

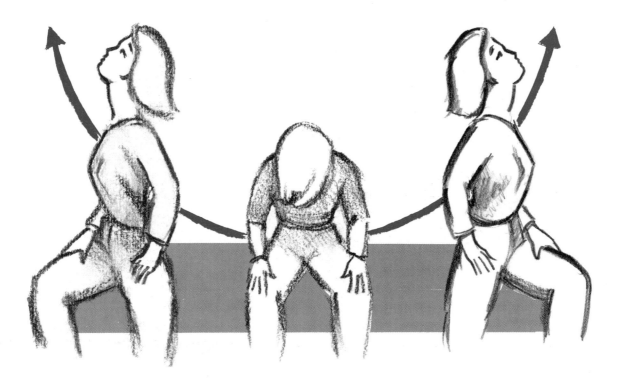

- This movement is smooth and continuous.
- Notice that when you turn to the right and look upward, your left hip rises a little. And when you turn to the left and look upward, your right hip rises a little.
- Notice that when you look upward, your shoulder blades move closer together. And when you look downward, your shoulder blades move farther apart.
- Arch your back as much as you can without feeling *any* strain.
- Round your back as much as you can without feeling *any* strain.

relax your entire body

let your body move freely

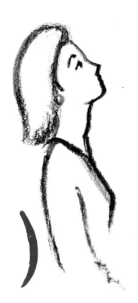

Measure your improvement: Lift your head and eyes to look upward while arching your back.

- When you look up, notice how much farther you can see without *any* strain!
- Feel your entire spine bending easily!
- Feel the difference!

And now, relax.

Feel how your weight is balanced, resting comfortably on your pelvic sitting bones. Notice that your posture is more upright. Your sitting posture has improved because the natural arches of your spine have been enhanced and restored.

You have completed **"A Healthy Spine."** When you stand up and walk around, feel the difference in your posture, flexibility, and ease of movement.

Enjoy the improvement!

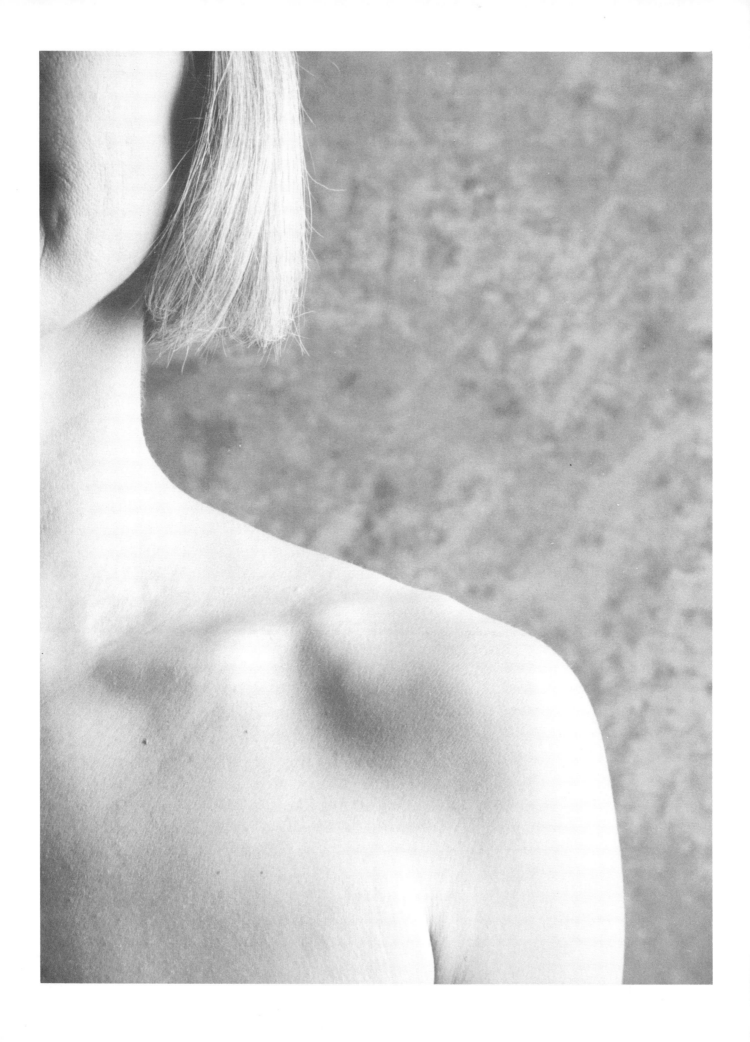

4 RELAXED SHOULDERS

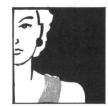

Mary P., a thirty-six-year-old Chicago homemaker, suffered shoulder tension, pain, and occasional numbness in the fingers of her right hand for over five years. Her family doctor prescribed rest and muscle relaxants—which helped initially—but eventually the pain returned and became chronic. By using the Relaxercise exercises, Mary learned how to relax her shoulders whenever they began to feel tense and, after only a few months, was completely pain free.

Our shoulder area is especially vulnerable to the development of muscular tension and discomfort. One of our body's most common responses to stress is to lift and tense our shoulders. This physical reaction is part of the well-known "fight-or-flight" reflex. Unfortunately, it is very easy to develop a habit of keeping our shoulders tense. Often, it is not until our shoulders are sore and stiff that we become aware of the tension held there.

The shoulder area is particularly susceptible to aches and pains when we spend long periods of time bending forward over desks, tables, machines, and so forth. Bending forward for long periods of time causes your upper back, neck, and shoulders to round and tighten. Unnecessary muscular tension in the shoulder area seriously restricts the flexibility of your neck, chest, arms, and back and has an adverse effect on your posture.

"Relaxed Shoulders" will help to restore the flexibility of your neck, chest, and back. You'll learn how to eliminate muscular tension in your shoulders—even if they have been chronically tense for many years.

RELAXED SHOULDERS

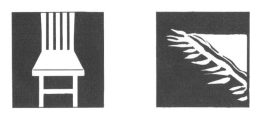

You will need either a hard or firmly cushioned chair or seat or an exercise mat or rug. Movements 1 to 10 will improve your **right** shoulder, movements 11 to 20 will improve your **left** shoulder.

Use the Relaxercise Keys

- **Go slowly.**

- **Make each movement small and easy.**

- **Relax as much as you can.**

- **Rest briefly after each movement.**

STARTING POSITIONS

Seated   Sit on the forward part of your chair or seat and rest your hands on your thighs. Rest your feet flat on the floor, shoulder width apart, directly below your knees.

Lying down   Lie on your left side with your left arm under your head and your right arm resting on your right side. Rest your right leg on top of your left leg. Bend both knees perpendicular to your pelvis. If you are uncomfortable, put a small pillow under your head. Your right arm remains lying on your right side throughout this part of the exercise.

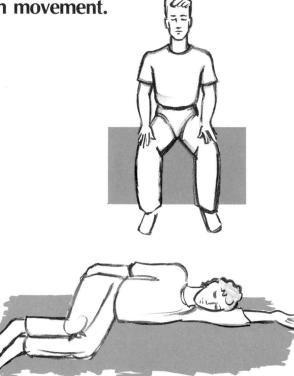

1

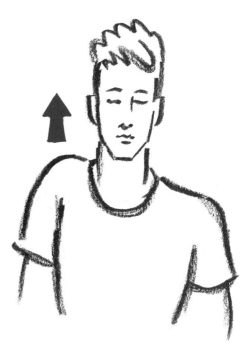

Very slowly, raise your right shoulder a little. Then return to the starting position and relax.

- Raise your shoulder without using your arm muscles. Your right arm can be passive and relaxed.
- Relax your neck, chest, and back.
- Breathe easily.
- Notice that the right side of your chest gets a little longer and the left side of your chest gets a little shorter.

2

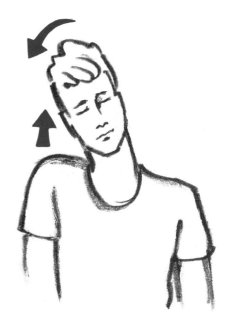

Simultaneously, tilt your head slowly to the right a little while raising your right shoulder. Your right ear and right shoulder will move toward each other. Then return to the starting position and relax.

- Don't turn your head—just **tilt** it while facing forward.
- Exhale as you do each movement.

after each movement, relax your shoulder completely

exhale as you do each movement

3 Just raise your right shoulder a little.

- Do you feel an improvement?
- Does your right shoulder feel more relaxed?

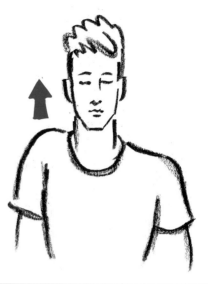

4 Very slowly, move your right shoulder downward a little. Then return to the starting position and relax.

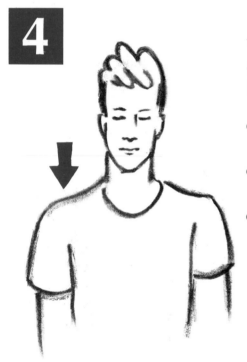

- Make each movement small, slow, and easy. Don't stretch or strain.
- Relax your right arm as much as possible.
- Notice that the ribs on your right side move closer together when you lower your right shoulder.

And now, rest for a moment.

- Feel how relaxed your right shoulder is!
- Does your right shoulder feel lower than your left shoulder?

relax your neck and shoulder

5

Very slowly move your right shoulder backward a little. Then return to the starting position and relax.

- Make each movement small and easy.
- Notice that your shoulder blade moves a little closer to your spine when you move your shoulder backward.

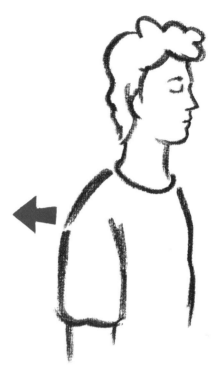

6

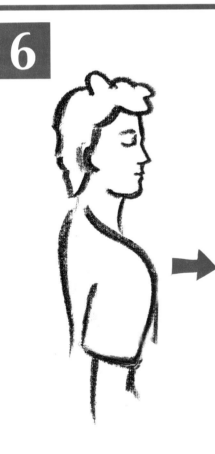

Slowly move your right shoulder forward a little. Then return to the starting position and relax.

- Notice that your shoulder blade moves away from your spine when your right shoulder moves forward.
- Do not use force. Your flexibility will increase automatically.

pause to rest after each movement

61

7 Simultaneously, move your right shoulder forward a little while turning your head slowly to the right. Then return to the starting position and rest.

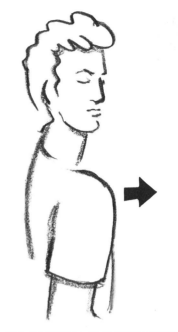

- Turn your head—don't tilt it.
- Notice that your chin and right shoulder are moving toward each other.
- Relax your neck and shoulder.
- If you are lying on your side, do not lift your head.

8 Again, move your right shoulder forward a little. Then return to the starting position and relax.

- Feel the improvement!
- Notice that your head and neck are turning spontaneously to the left a little.

9

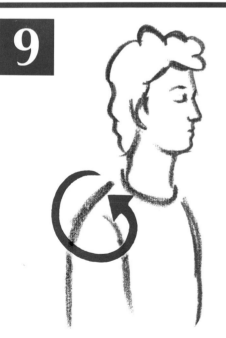

Make a relaxed, circular movement with your right shoulder: Slowly raise your right shoulder a little, rotate it gently back, down, forward, and up again.

- Rest after every few rotations.
- Do not stretch. Your flexibility will increase automatically.
- Make each circular movement relaxed and easy.
- To make the movement smooth and even, make the circle smaller.

let your body move freely

10

Reverse the direction of the circular movement: Slowly raise your right shoulder a little. Then rotate it gently forward, down, back, and up again.

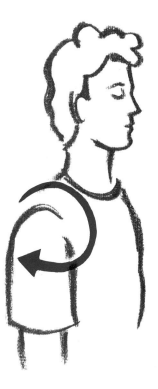

- Rest after every few rotations.
- To make each movement smooth and even, make the circle smaller and slower.
- Notice how rotating your shoulder makes your head, neck, chest, back, and pelvis move a little.

And now, rest.

- If you are lying down, rest on your back.
- Notice how different your right shoulder feels from your left shoulder!
- Feel the difference in your face, neck, chest, and pelvis.

Stand up and walk around. Feel the difference between your right and left shoulders.

Feel the difference!

To improve your left shoulder
continue with movements 11 through 20.

The following movements will improve your *left* shoulder.

STARTING POSITIONS

Seated Sit on the forward part of your chair or seat, and rest your hands on your thighs. Rest your feet flat on the floor, shoulder width apart, directly below your knees.

Lying down Lie on your right side, with your right arm under your head and your left arm resting on your left side. Rest your left leg on top of your right leg. Bend your knees perpendicular to your pelvis. If you are uncomfortable, place a small pillow under your head.

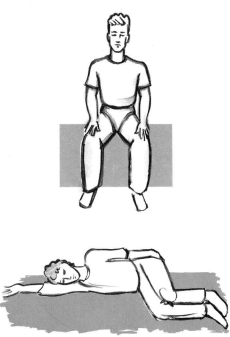

11

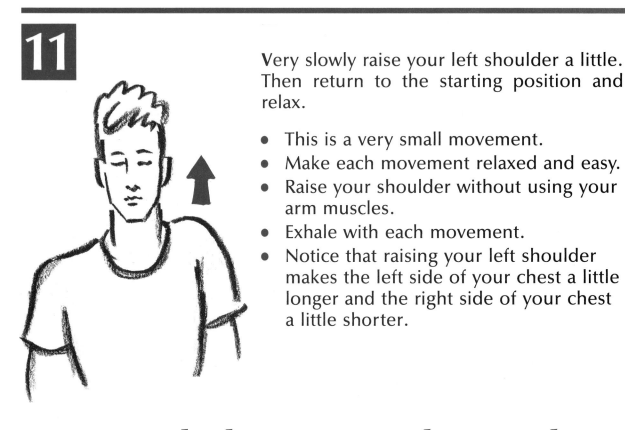

Very slowly raise your left shoulder a little. Then return to the starting position and relax.

- This is a very small movement.
- Make each movement relaxed and easy.
- Raise your shoulder without using your arm muscles.
- Exhale with each movement.
- Notice that raising your left shoulder makes the left side of your chest a little longer and the right side of your chest a little shorter.

go slowly so your muscles can relax

relax your neck, back, stomach and legs

12 Simultaneously, tilt your head to the left a little while raising your left shoulder. Your left ear and left shoulder will move toward each other. Then return to the starting position and relax.

- Don't turn your head. Tilt it while facing forward.
- Exhale as you do each movement.

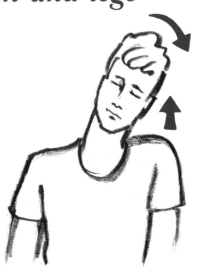

13

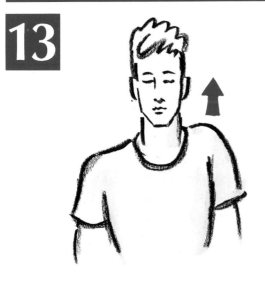

Again, just raise your left shoulder a little. Then return to the starting position and relax.

- Can you feel an improvement?
- Does your left shoulder feel more relaxed already?

14 Very slowly move your left shoulder downward a little. Then return to the starting position and relax.

- Make each movement small and slight.
- Notice that lowering your left shoulder makes the ribs on your left side move closer together.

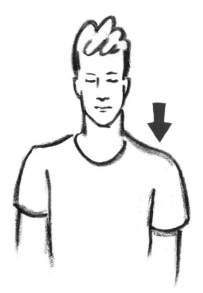

pause to rest after each movement

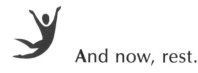

And now, rest.

- Feel how relaxed your left shoulder is.
- Is your left shoulder lower than it was a few minutes ago?

15

Very slowly, move your left shoulder backward a little. Then return to the starting position and rest.

- Make each movement small and easy.
- Do not use force. Your flexibility will increase automatically.
- Relax your left shoulder and arm as much as possible.
- Relax your chest and lower back.
- Notice that your shoulder blade moves closer to your spine when your shoulder moves backward.

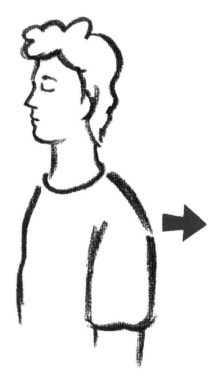

don't stretch or strain

make each movement small and easy

16

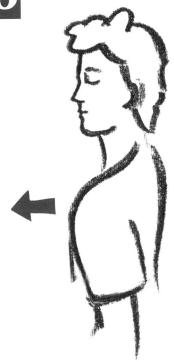

Very slowly move your left shoulder forward a little. Then return to the starting position and rest.

- Relax your shoulder completely between each movement.
- Notice that your shoulder blade moves away from your spine when your left shoulder moves forward.
- Relax your arm, neck, and chest.

17

Simultaneously, move your left shoulder forward a little, while turning your head slowly to the left. Then return to the starting position and rest.

- Notice that your chin and left shoulder are moving toward each other.
- If you are lying on your side, don't lift your head.

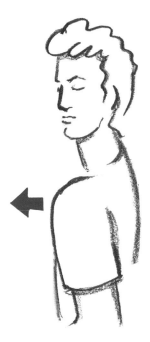

use as little muscular effort as possible

18

Again, just move your left shoulder forward a little. Then return to the starting position and rest.

- Notice that your head, neck, and chest are now turning to the right a little when you do this movement.

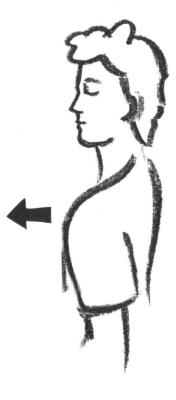

19

Make a relaxed circular movement with your left shoulder: Slowly raise your left shoulder a little, and rotate it back, down, forward, and up again.

- Rest after every few rotations.
- To make the movement smoother, make the circle smaller.
- Relax your arm as much as possible.
- Notice that rotating your shoulder makes your head, neck, chest, back, and pelvis move a little.
- Breathe freely.

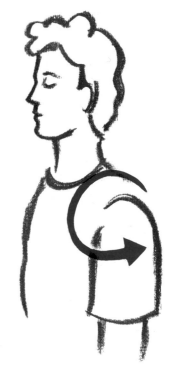

let your body move freely

20

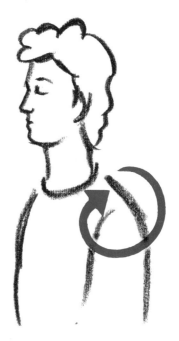

Reverse the direction of the circular movement: Very slowly raise your left shoulder a little, and rotate it gently, forward, down, back, and up again.

- Make each movement relaxed and easy.
- Notice how when you changed the direction, the movement of your head, neck, chest, and pelvis changed direction, too.

And now, rest.

If you are lying down, rest on your back. Notice how relaxed your entire left side feels. Feel the difference in your face, neck, chest, and pelvis!

You have completed **"Relaxed Shoulders."** Stand up and walk around. Notice how comfortable your shoulders are. Do you feel taller? Notice how relaxed and light your entire body feels.

Enjoy the improvement!

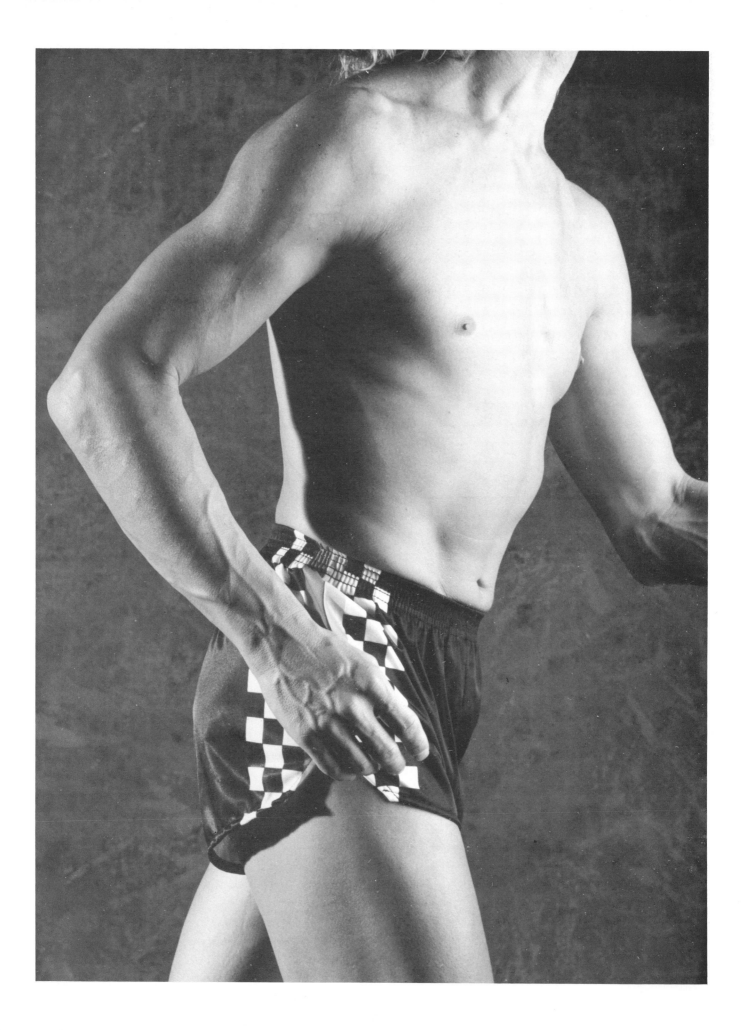

5 YOUR POWER CENTER

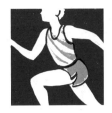

Bill A., a prosperous forty-eight-year-old dentist, was not able to enjoy his success. Bill suffered chronic neck pain and a herniated lumbar disc, both the result of constantly bending over to work on his patients. After two years of trying conventional back programs, acupuncture, and pain-relieving drugs, Bill's orthopedist recommended back surgery. A second orthopedist referred Bill to us. With Relaxercise, Bill gradually became free of pain and learned how to bend forward at work without jeopardizing his back or neck.

The largest and most powerful muscles of your body are the ones connected to your pelvis. Without their effective participation, you would not be able to do even such basic activities as standing, walking, running, pushing, pulling, lifting, or anything else requiring physical power. The muscles connected to your pelvis are vital to the support of your lower back and protect your back from strain and injury.

Due to our sedentary life-styles, these particular muscles often become tense, weak and consequently, less effective. When this happens, your body is like a car engine running on only half its cylinders. Smaller and weaker muscles have to compensate by working harder than they should; your hip joints tighten and become restricted, your lower back is strained, and your muscles and ligaments experience dangerous amounts of wear and tear.

"Your Power Center" will help you make remarkable improvements in the flexibility and strength of your hip joints and lower back. This exercise will also mobilize the powerful muscles connected to your pelvis so they can work efficiently—as nature intended, and you will feel immediate improvements in your posture and vitality.

YOUR POWER CENTER

You will need a hard or firmly cushioned chair or seat.

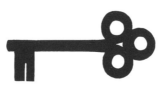

Use the Relaxercise Keys

- **Go slowly.**

- **Make each movement small and easy.**

- **Relax as much as you can.**

- **Rest briefly after each movement.**

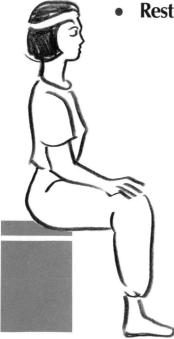

STARTING POSITION
Sit on the forward part of your chair and rest your hands on your thighs.
Rest your feet flat on the floor, shoulder width apart, directly below your knees.

1

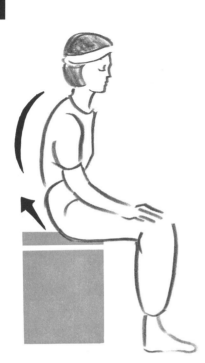

Slowly tilt your pelvis backward a little so your lower back rounds slightly. Then return to the starting position and rest.

- Make the movement very small. Just slowly tilt your pelvis back **slightly**.
- Relax your neck, shoulders, chest, stomach, and legs.
- Notice that when you tilt your pelvis back, your weight shifts from your pelvic sitting bones to the area near your tailbone. When you return to the starting position, your weight shifts forward to your sitting bones again.
- Notice that your body gets a little shorter when your pelvis is tilted back.
- Exhale as you do each movement.

2

Slowly tilt your pelvis forward a little so your lower back arches slightly. Then return to the starting position and rest.

- Relax your stomach, back, and legs.
- Feel your weight moving toward the front of your pelvic sitting bones.
- When you tilt your pelvis forward, your body gets a little taller and more upright.
- Do not tilt your entire upper body forward—just tilt your pelvis **slightly**.
- Exhale as you do each movement.

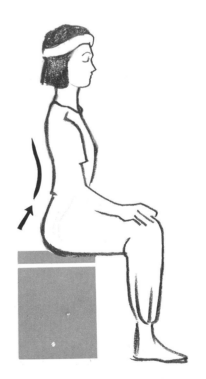

pause to rest after each movement

3

Slowly tilt your pelvis forward a little so your back arches slightly and your body gets a little taller. Then slowly tilt your pelvis backward a little so your back rounds slightly and your body gets a little shorter.

- Slowly rock your pelvis back and forth.
- When you round your back, your shoulders move forward slightly. And, when you arch your back, your shoulders move back slightly.
- Notice how your head moves up and down a little as you tilt your pelvis back and forth.
- Relax your chest so it can move freely. Notice how your chest rises when you tilt your pelvis forward and sinks when you tilt your pelvis backward.
- Notice that your entire spine is moving a little.
- Feel your weight shifting back and forth on your pelvic sitting bones.
- Relax your entire body as much as you can.

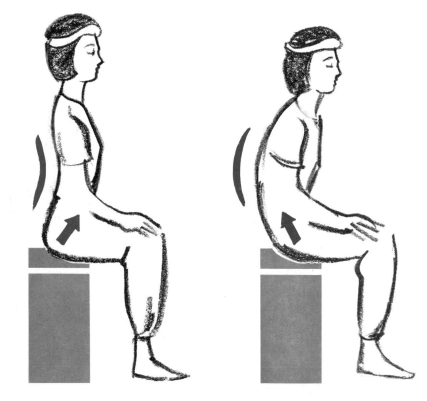

relax . . . your flexibility will increase automatically

4

Slowly tilt your pelvis toward your left knee a little so your weight shifts toward the forward part of your left buttock. Then return to the starting position and rest.

- Keep your feet flat on the floor.
- When your pelvis tilts toward your left knee, the weight of your right buttock lifts a little and your lower back arches slightly.
- With each movement your head moves a little to the left and your body gets a little taller.
- Notice how your left shoulder is moving back a little, and your right shoulder is moving forward a little.

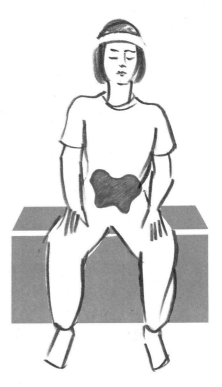

5

Tilt your pelvis toward your right knee a little so your weight shifts toward the forward part of your right buttock. Then return to the starting position and rest.

- When your pelvis tilts toward your right knee, the weight of your left buttock lifts a little and your lower back arches.
- As you do the movement, your head moves a little to the right and your body gets a little taller.
- Does it feel easier to tilt your pelvis to the right, or does it feel easier to tilt it to the left?
- Notice how your right shoulder is moving back a little, and your left shoulder is moving forward a little.

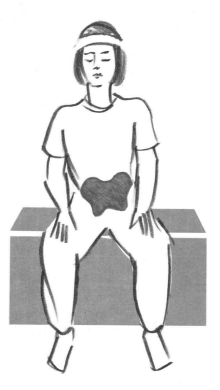

repeat each movement 4 to 8 times

6 Slowly tilt your pelvis toward your left knee so your weight shifts to your left buttock. Return to the starting position and then slowly tilt your pelvis toward your right knee so your weight shifts to your right buttock.

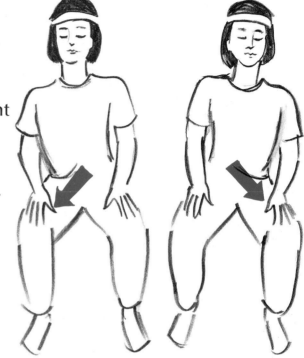

- When your pelvis tilts toward your left knee, the ribs on your right side move closer together and you get a little taller.
- When your pelvis tilts toward your right knee, the ribs on your left side move closer together and you get a little taller.
- Notice how as your pelvis moves, your head moves, too.
- Try to make the movement on both sides equally smooth and easy.

FOR MOVEMENTS 7 TO 14:

Imagine that you are sitting on a small, flat, round, clock dial painted on the seat of your chair.

When you tilt your pelvis back, you are tilting toward **6 o'clock**.

When you tilt your pelvis forward, you are tilting toward **12 o'clock**.

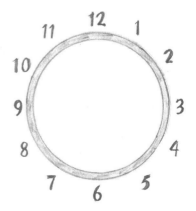

When you tilt your pelvis to the left, you are tilting toward **9 o'clock**.

When you tilt your pelvis to the right, you are tilting toward **3 o'clock**.

use as little effort as possible

7 Tilt your pelvis back to 6 o'clock so your lower back rounds. Then slowly roll your pelvis in a small arc toward the right to 3 o'clock so your back curves a little. Then slowly return, moving along the arc until you reach 6 o'clock again and your lower back is rounded. Move your pelvis back and forth slowly between 6 o'clock and 3 o'clock. At 3 o'clock and 6 o'clock, pause to rest for a moment.

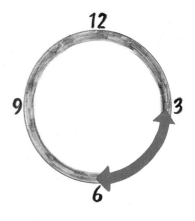

- Notice that at the 3 o'clock position, your weight is entirely on your right buttock.
- Relax your entire body as much as possible.

8 Tilt your pelvis forward to 12 o'clock so your lower back arches and your abdomen moves forward. Then slowly roll your pelvis in a small arc toward the right, to 3 o'clock, so your back curves a little. Then return, moving slowly through the arc until you reach 12 o'clock and your lower back is arched. Move your pelvis back and forth slowly between 12 o'clock and 3 o'clock. At 3 o'clock and 12 o'clock, pause to rest for a moment.

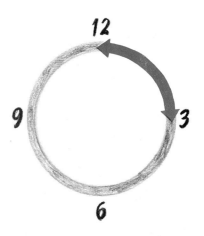

- Notice that at the 3 o'clock position, the arch of your lower back has diminished.
- Relax your back and stomach muscles, and let your head and neck move freely.

go slowly so your muscles can relax

make each movement slow, easy and comfortable

9

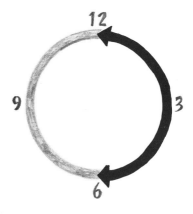

Very slowly roll your pelvis in an arc from 12 o'clock to 6 o'clock along the right side of the clock. Start at 12 o'clock, with your back arched. Roll your pelvis slowly to the right, through 1, 2, 3, 4, and 5 o'clock, to 6 o'clock, where your lower back is rounded. Then return, moving slowly along the arc, until you reach 12 o'clock again. Move your pelvis back and forth slowly between 12 o'clock and 6 o'clock. At 12 o'clock and 6 o'clock, pause to rest.

- This is a continuous movement.
- Make the arc smooth and easy by relaxing as much as possible.
- Feel your weight rolling along each hour of the arc.
- Notice how your body gets a little taller as you reach 12 o'clock and a little shorter as you reach 6 o'clock.
- Feel your head, chest, and back following the movement of your pelvis.

And now, rest for a moment.

- Notice that your right side is more relaxed than your left side!
- Notice that you are sitting with more of your weight on your right pelvic sitting bone.

feel the difference!

10

Tilt your pelvis back to 6 o'clock so your lower back rounds. Then slowly roll your pelvis in a small arc to the left—to 9 o'clock—so your back curves a little. Then return . . . move back along the arc until you reach 6 o'clock and your lower back is rounded. Move your pelvis back and forth slowly between 6 o'clock and 9 o'clock. At 6 o'clock and 9 o'clock, pause to rest.

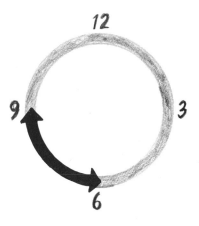

- Notice that at the 9 o'clock position, your weight is entirely on your left buttock.
- Relax your entire body as much as possible.
- Notice that as you move toward 9 o'clock, your stomach moves forward and your body gets a little taller.

11

Tilt your pelvis forward to 12 o'clock so your lower back arches and your abdomen moves forward. Then slowly roll your pelvis in a small arc toward the left to 9 o'clock so your back curves a little. Then return, moving back along the arc until you reach 12 o'clock again and your lower back is arched. Move your pelvis back and forth slowly between 12 o'clock and 9 o'clock. At 9 o'clock and 12 o'clock, pause to rest.

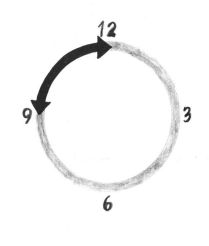

- Notice that at the 9 o'clock position, the arch of your lower back has diminished.
- Relax your back and stomach muscles.

rest briefly between each movement

12 Very slowly roll your pelvis in an arc from 12 o'clock to 6 o'clock, along the left-hand side of the clock. Start at 12 o'clock, with your back arched, and slowly roll your pelvis to the left, moving through 11, 10, 9, 8, and 7 o'clock, to 6 o'clock, with your lower back rounded. Then return, moving back along the arc until you again reach 12 o'clock. Move your pelvis back and forth slowly between 12 o'clock and 6 o'clock. At 12 o'clock and 6 o'clock, pause to rest.

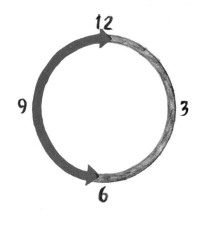

- This is a continuous movement.
- Make the movement smoother by relaxing.
- Feel your weight rolling along each hour of the arc.
- Notice how your body gets a little taller as you reach 12 o'clock and a little shorter as you reach 6 o'clock.
- Feel your head, chest, and back following the movement of your pelvis.
- Relax your neck, back, stomach, and legs.

13 Very slowly tilt your pelvis forward to 12 o'clock. Then slowly roll your pelvis in a clockwise direction around the dial of the clock. Pass through each hour, making a continuous circular movement.

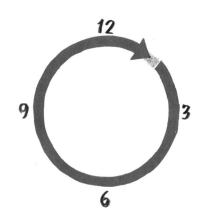

- Go slowly.
- To make the movement easier, make the circle smaller.
- Notice how your head and chest are also making circular movements.

let your body move freely

14 Tilt your pelvis forward to 12 o'clock and then slowly roll your pelvis in a counter-clockwise direction around the dial of the clock. Slowly pass through each hour, making a continuous circular movement.

- Relax your entire body.
- Notice that your head and chest are making a counterclockwise circular movement.
- Does the counterclockwise circular movement feel different from the clockwise circular movement?

And now, rest.

Notice how **little** muscular effort you require to sit upright. Feel how easily you can shift your pelvis to the right, to the left, forward, and backward. Feel how your weight is balanced evenly on your sitting bones.

You have completed **"Your Power Center."** When you stand up and walk around, notice the new flexibility in your hips, back, and legs. Notice how much more relaxed and taller you feel.

ADVANCED VERSION

"Your Power Center" may also be done while sitting on the floor, with the soles of your feet together, your hands resting on the floor behind you, with your fingers pointed away from your body. Rest on your back whenever you wish. Do not attempt the advanced version of "Your Power Center" until you have done the exercise at least twice while seated in a chair.

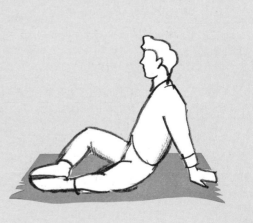

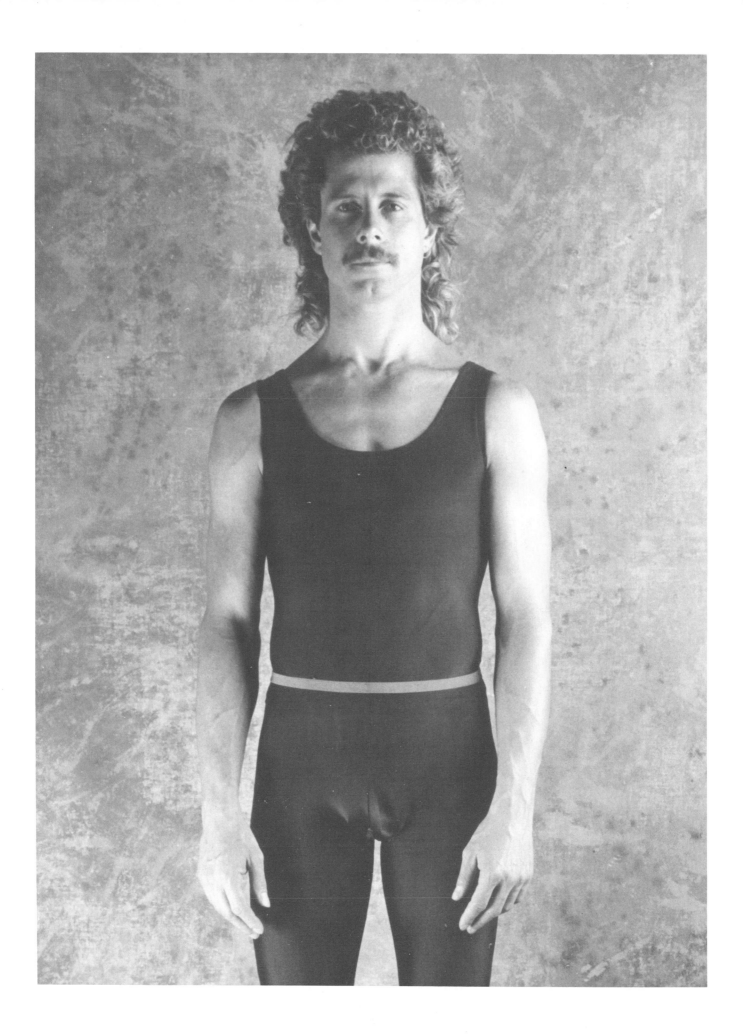

6

ALIGNING YOUR BODY

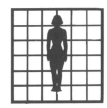

Virginia C., a forty-eight-year-old resident of New York City, was concerned with the way her body was changing. She noticed that her posture had deteriorated; her joints often ached and the flexibility and freedom of movement she used to enjoy had disappeared. Her doctor told her that these problems were unavoidable aspects of getting older. However, by using Relaxercise, Virginia was able to restore her posture, regain almost all of her flexibility, and enjoy a renewed sense of youthful vitality.

"Aligning Your Body" will improve one of your spine's most important movements—bending *sideways*. Every day your spine bends to the left and right, thousands of times. Even when you are sitting in a chair and your body is relatively inactive, your spine makes countless slight bending movements as you change your position, reach for a pen, use the telephone, and so on.

Bending sideways is a surprisingly complex movement. Each time you bend to the right, for example, the right side of your body becomes a little shorter, the left side of your body becomes a little longer, and your body must work to maintain its balance.

Your spine's ability to bend sideways can become limited without your even realizing it. When this happens, the muscular and skeletal alignment of your body suffers. The muscles along one side of your neck, chest, and back become chronically tense and are often painfully stiff. Over time, asymmetrical alignment can become a postural habit, which makes you especially susceptible to muscle and joint discomfort and neck and low back pain. With poor alignment, even simple movements involve more muscular exertion and stress than is really necessary.

"Aligning Your Body" will improve your alignment, flexibility, and ease of movement. When your body is properly aligned, your neck and lower back will be instantly relieved and more comfortable, and you will enjoy greater freedom of movement.

ALIGNING YOUR BODY

You will need a hard or firmly cushioned chair or seat.

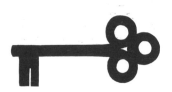

Use the Relaxercise Keys

- **Go slowly.**

- **Make each movement small and easy.**

- **Relax as much as you can.**

- **Rest briefly after each movement.**

STARTING POSITION
Sit on the forward edge of your chair or seat
and rest your hands on your thighs.
Rest your feet flat on the floor, shoulder
width apart, directly below your knees.

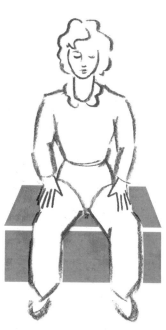

1

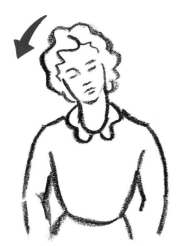

Very slowly tilt your head toward your right shoulder a little. Then return to the starting position and relax.

- Tilt your head to the right, **without** turning it. Continue facing forward as you tilt your head.
- Make each movement very small and easy.
- Relax your neck, shoulders, and chest.
- Don't stretch or strain. Your flexibility will increase all by itself.
- Notice how as you tilt your head to the right, the ribs on your right side move closer together.
- Exhale as you do each movement.

2

Lift the weight of your right buttock slightly. Simply transfer your weight onto your left buttock so you can easily lift the weight of your right buttock. Then return to the starting position and rest.

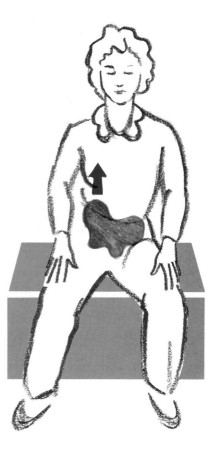

- This is a very slight movement. Your right buttock does **not** need to lift off the seat.
- Make each movement slow and small.
- Notice how as you lift your right buttock, your right foot presses the floor gently.
- Relax your right leg, shoulder, and stomach.
- Notice that when you lift your right buttock, the ribs on your right side move closer together and your head tilts a little to the right.

pause to rest after each movement

3

Simultaneously, tilt your head toward your right shoulder while lifting the weight of your right buttock slightly. Then return to the starting position and rest.

- Make each movement smooth and continuous.
- Notice that your right ear and right hip move toward each other, while your left ear and left hip move farther apart.
- Your spine is bending like a letter C.

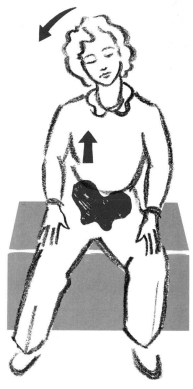

4

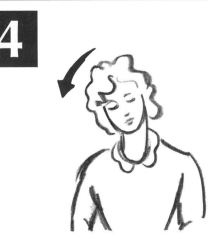

Again, tilt your head toward your right shoulder a few times. Return to the starting position between each movement.

Notice how the right side of your neck and chest are already more flexible and relaxed.

And now, rest for a moment.

- Does the right side of your neck and back feel a little longer and more relaxed than the left side?
- Is more of your weight on your right buttock and sitting bone?

repeat each movement 4 to 8 times

5 Very slowly tilt your head toward your left shoulder. Then return to the starting position and rest.

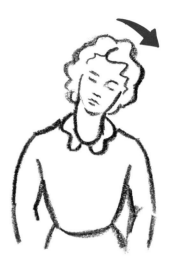

- Don't turn your head. Just **tilt** your head while facing forward.
- Make this movement slight and comfortable. Don't stretch or strain.
- Notice how as you tilt your head to the left, the ribs on your left side move closer together.
- As you tilt your head, do you feel your weight beginning to shift toward your right buttock?
- Exhale as you do each movement.

6

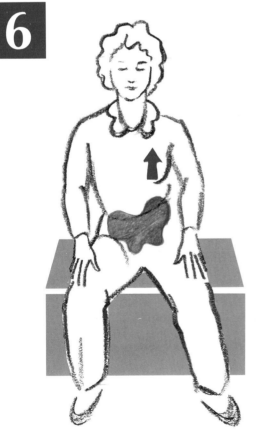

Very slowly lift the weight of your left buttock slightly. Simply transfer your weight to your right buttock so you can easily lift the weight of your left buttock a little. Then return to the starting position and relax.

- This is a small, easy movement. Your right buttock does **not** need to lift off the seat.
- Use as little muscular effort as possible.
- Notice how as you lift your left buttock, your left foot presses against the floor gently and your head and chest bend a little to the left.
- Feel your weight shift from your left buttock to your right buttock.

relax your neck, back, stomach and legs

7

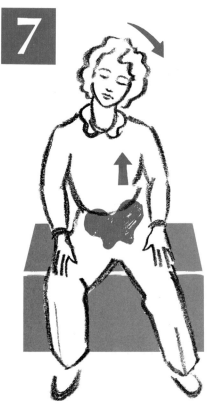

Simultaneously, tilt your head toward your left shoulder while lifting the weight of your left buttock very slightly. Then return to the starting position and relax.

- Use as little effort as possible, so your spine and chest can move freely.
- Relax your neck, arms, shoulders, chest, lower back, and legs.
- Notice that your left ear and left hip are moving toward each other, while your right ear and right hip are moving farther apart.
- Your spine is bending like a letter C.

8

Again, tilt your head toward your left shoulder. Then return to the starting position.

- Notice how your flexibility and ease of movement have already increased.

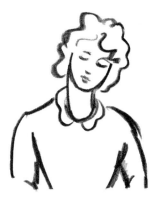

 And now, rest.

- Feel the left side of your neck and lower back becoming more relaxed.
- Notice that your weight is more evenly distributed between both of your pelvic sitting bones. When your weight is equally distributed, the muscular stress of sitting for long periods of time is significantly reduced.

use as little effort as possible

go slowly so your muscles can relax

9

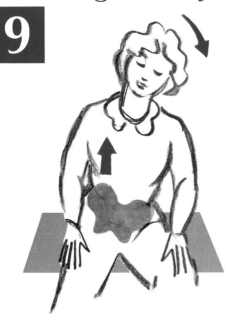

Simultaneously, tilt your head toward your left shoulder while lifting the weight of your right buttock very slightly. Then return to the starting position and rest.

- Go slowly.
- Breathe freely.
- Your spine is making a shape like a letter S.

10

Simply tilt your head to the right. Then return to the starting position.

- Feel your entire body bending to the right.
- Feel how your right hip is lifting.
- Has your flexibility improved even more?

11

Simultaneously, tilt your head to the right while lifting the weight of your left buttock very slightly. Then return to the starting position and rest.

- Breathe freely.
- Your spine is making a shape like a letter S:

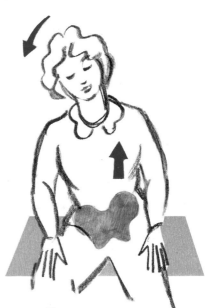

make each movement slight and easy

12

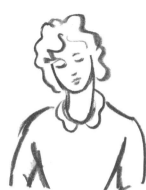

Simply tilt your head to the left.

* Feel how your neck, chest, and back are bending more easily!
* Feel the improvement!

13

Simultaneously, tilt your right ear toward your right shoulder, while lifting your right buttock very slightly. Then return—but move *through* the starting position without stopping—tilt your left ear toward your left shoulder, while lifting your left buttock.

* Alternate 4 to 8 times.
* Make each movement smooth and continuous.
* Go slowly, so each movement can be more relaxed.
* Does your body bend more easily to the left or to the right?
* Relax your neck, shoulders, chest, and lower back so both sides can bend more freely.
* Notice how your weight shifts from side to side.

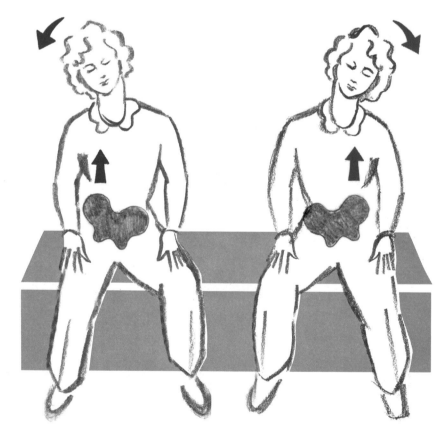

pause to rest after every few movements

make each movement slow and comfortable

14 **K**eep your head and eyes facing forward, and continue alternately lifting your right and left buttocks.

- Rock your pelvis from side to side, without tilting your neck and head.
- Relax your legs, stomach, and shoulders.
- Feel your lower spine bending.

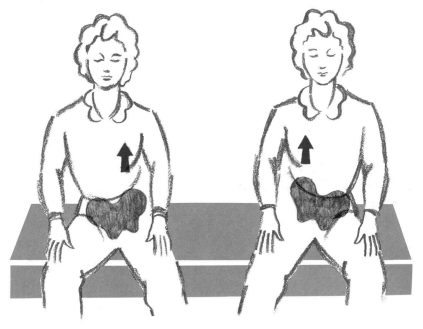

---

15 Measure your improvement: Tilt your head to the right and left a few times.

- Feel how your flexibility has increased!
- Feel the difference!

And now, rest.

Notice that your weight is now evenly balanced between your right and left pelvic sitting bones, and your sitting posture has improved. This will protect your neck and back from stress and strain.

You have completed **"Aligning Your Body."** When you stand up and walk around, notice the difference in your posture and ease of movement!

Enjoy your improvement!

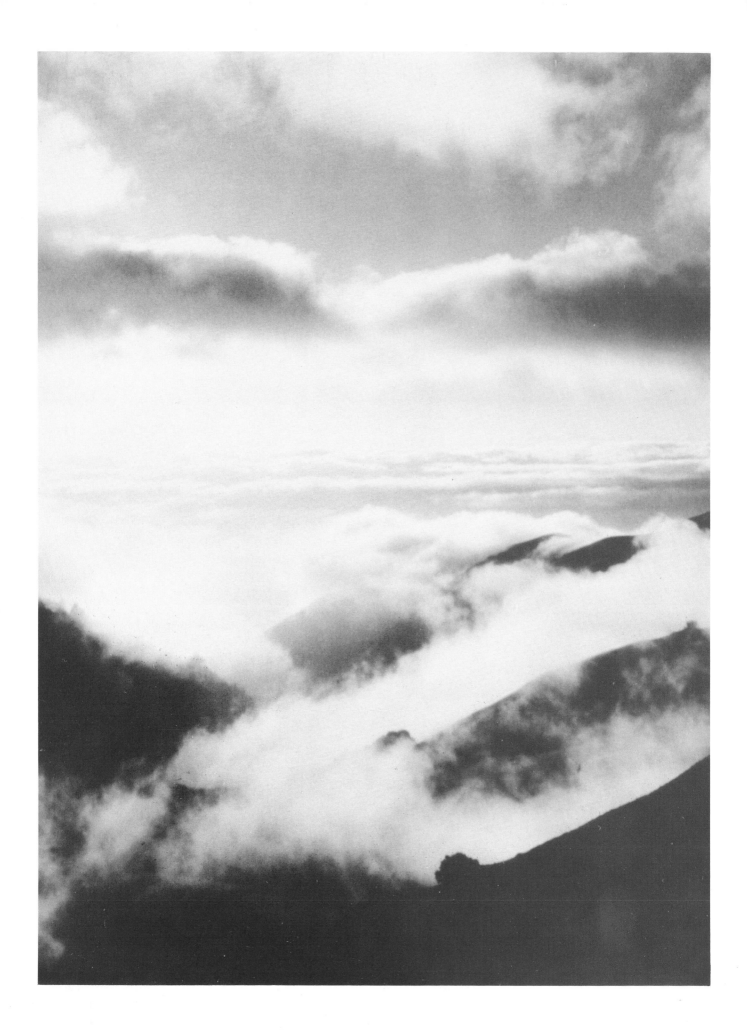

7 FULL BREATHING

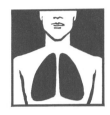

John D., a sixty-eight-year-old retired machinist, had been a resident of Los Angeles for over forty years. When John first came to see us, he suffered from shortness of breath, could not go outdoors on smoggy days, and was unable to engage in any sort of active exercise. After using Relaxercise exercises for four weeks, John's breathing capacity had increased by nearly 50 percent, and he was able to walk up to a mile a day, comfortably.

Living is not possible without breathing. We breathe every moment of our lives, inhaling and exhaling over twenty thousand times each day. But we hardly ever stop to think about our breathing. Our breathing is regulated by our brain and adjusts automatically to every change in our activity and emotion. Whether we are fearful or confident, relaxed or excited, joyous or angry, our breathing alters accordingly, becoming either quicker or slower, deeper or more shallow.

We live in a fast-paced modern world in which tension and stress are hard to avoid. One of our first responses to stress is to hold our breath and tighten our chest. Constricted breathing can easily become a habit. In fact, your breathing can become so restricted that before you know it, you are using only 50 percent of your natural lung capacity. Over time, habits of restricted breathing can drain your vitality and have an adverse effect on your health, posture, and flexibility.

There are two basic human breathing patterns. In one, the abdomen expands as you inhale; this is called "diaphragmatic breathing." In the other, the abdomen is drawn in, and the chest expands while inhaling. This is called "paradoxical breathing." These are both natural and normal ways to breathe and vary according to your activity.

"Full Breathing" will show you how to quickly increase your lung capacity and achieve relaxed, stress-free breathing.

FULL BREATHING

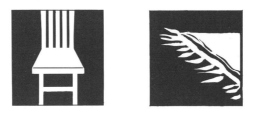

You will need a hard, or firmly cushioned chair or seat. For movements 1–6, you can also use an exercise mat or rug.

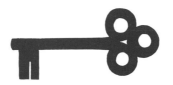

Use the Relaxercise Keys

- **Go slowly.**

- **Make each movement small and easy.**

- **Relax as much as you can.**

- **Rest briefly after each movement.**

Note: This entire exercise can be done either seated in a chair, or, you can do movements 1 through 6 while lying on your back. **Movements 7 through 13 must be done while seated in a chair.**

STARTING POSITIONS
Seated   Sit on the forward part of your chair or seat. Rest your hands on your thighs. Your feet should rest flat on the floor, shoulder width apart, directly below your knees.

Lying down   Lie on your back on a cushioned mat or rug and rest your arms comfortably by your sides. Bend your knees and rest your feet on the floor, shoulder width apart, directly below your knees.

repeat each movement 4 to 8 times

1 When you inhale (breathe in), slowly draw in your lower abdomen. Then exhale (breathe out) normally.

Your lower abdomen is the area between your belly button and your pubic bone.

- Don't breathe more deeply than usual.
- Feel your chest expanding as you inhale.
- Follow the movement of air as it passes through your nose and fills your chest.
- Relax your face, jaw, neck, shoulders, and legs.

---

2 Inhale normally, but while exhaling, slowly push the air down so your lower abdomen expands, becoming rounder and larger.

- Rest your hands on your lower abdomen and feel it expanding.
- Notice that when you exhale, your chest gets smaller and flatter.
- When you exhale and expand your lower abdomen, does one side of your abdomen expand more than the other?

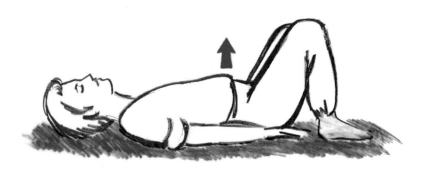

rest and breathe normally between each movement

alternate slowly

3 While inhaling, slowly draw in your lower abdomen and expand your chest. While exhaling, slowly expand your lower abdomen and let your chest flatten.

- Make each movement as smooth as possible.
- Go slowly so you can relax your shoulders, stomach, and legs.
- As you breathe in and out, feel the see-saw movement of your chest and abdomen.
- Notice how your chest expands in all directions: forward, backward, left, and right.

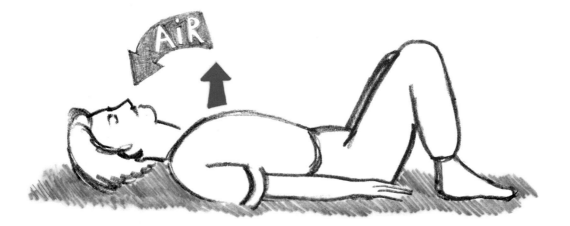

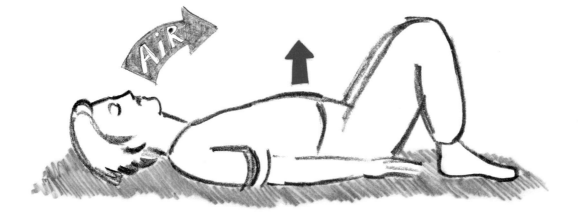

go slowly . . .

4

While inhaling, slowly draw in your lower abdomen and try to breathe into the right side of your chest. While exhaling, push the air down and into the left side of your lower abdomen.

- Note: this is a diagonal, see-saw movement.
- As you inhale, pay attention to the right side of your chest.
- As you exhale, pay attention to the left side of your lower abdomen.
- Put your hands on your lower abdomen so you can feel the left side expanding more than the right.

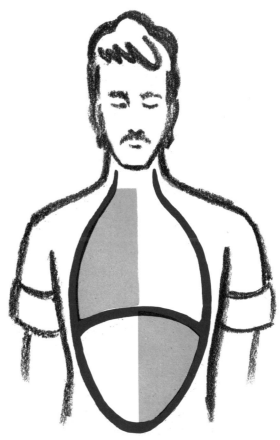

And now, rest.

- Feel the difference between the right and left sides of your chest.
- Feel the difference between the right and left sides of your lower abdomen.

pause to rest after each movement

make each movement slow and easy

5

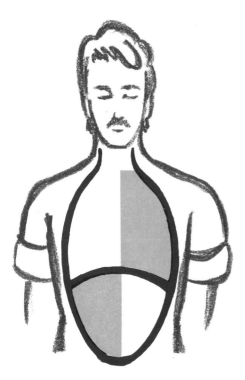

While inhaling, slowly draw in your lower abdomen and breathe into the left side of your chest. While exhaling, push the air down and into the right side of your lower abdomen.

- Feel the slight diagonal movement from your left shoulder to your right hip.
- Relax your entire body as much as possible.
- Rest your hands on your lower abdomen and feel it expanding.
- As you inhale, pay attention to the left side of your chest.
- As you exhale, pay attention to the right side of your lower abdomen.

6

While inhaling, slowly draw in your entire lower abdomen and let your chest expand. While exhaling, slowly expand your entire lower abdomen and let your chest flatten.

- Notice that your chest and abdomen are expanding more easily.
- Notice how as you exhale, your head lowers slightly, and as you inhale, your head rises slightly.

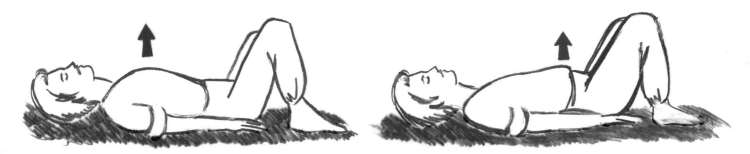

relax your entire body

repeat each movement 4 to 8 times

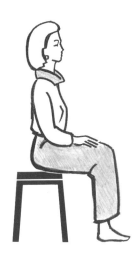

NOTE: The concluding series of movements must be done while seated. Sit on the forward part of a hard or firmly cushioned chair. Rest your hands on your thighs and rest your feet flat on the floor, shoulder width apart, directly below your knees.

7

Let your head hang down so your chin rests close to your chest. Then, while inhaling, slowly draw your lower abdomen in and expand your chest. While exhaling, slowly expand your lower abdomen and let your chest flatten.

- Notice that when you exhale, your entire body sinks down a little, and when you inhale, your entire body rises a little.

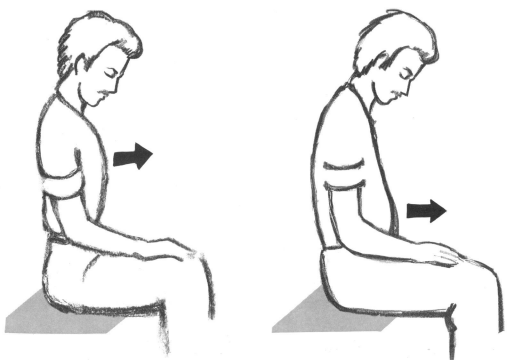

relax your neck and shoulders

breathe normally between each movement

8

While inhaling, slowly draw in your lower abdomen and lift your head to look up. While exhaling, slowly expand your lower abdomen and lower your head to look down.

- Your chest rises and lowers as your head moves up and down.
- Feel your spine moving. When you inhale, your back arches, and when you exhale, your back rounds.

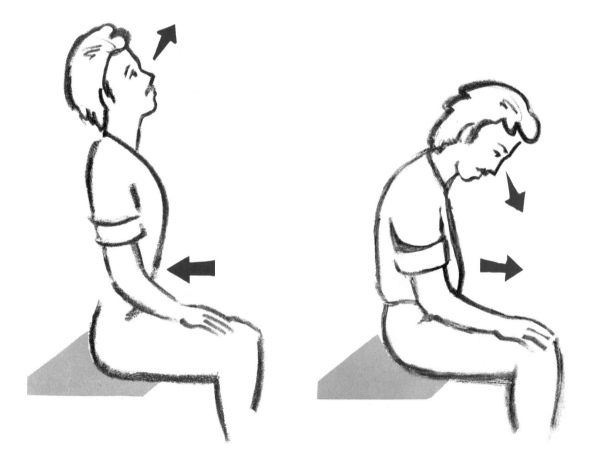

don't stretch or strain

9 For the next movement, embrace yourself gently. Cross your left arm over your chest and put your left hand over or near the lower ribs on your right side. Cross your right arm over your left arm and put your right hand under your left elbow near the lower ribs on your left side. Don't stretch!

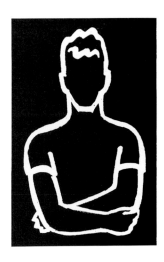

While inhaling, simultaneously draw in your lower abdomen, expand your chest, lift your head to look up, and arch your back. While exhaling, simultaneously expand your lower abdomen, let your chest flatten, lower your head to look down, and round your back.

- Relax your face, shoulders, chest, stomach, and legs.
- Notice how embracing yourself limits the movement of your chest.
- Feel the slight rocking movement of your lower back and pelvis.

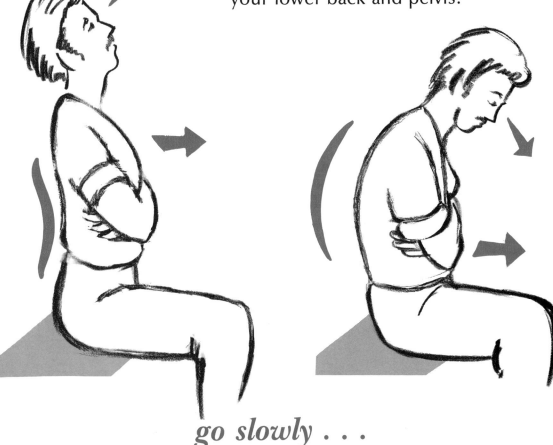

go slowly . . .

relax your entire body

10 Reverse the position of your arms: Embrace yourself, with your left arm crossing over your right arm.

While inhaling, simultaneously draw in your lower abdomen, expand your chest, lift your head to look up, and arch your back. While exhaling, simultaneously expand your lower abdomen, let your chest flatten, lower your head to look down, and round your back.

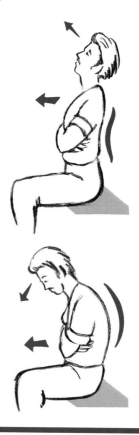

- Feel your chest rising and lowering with the movement of your head.
- The more you arch your back, the more your chest rises.

And now, rest.

- Feel your chest expanding in all directions more easily!
- Your sitting posture has improved and is more upright!
- Notice how relaxed your breathing is!

11 While inhaling, slowly draw in your lower abdomen and lift your head to look up. While exhaling, slowly expand your lower abdomen and lower your head to look down.

- Feel how your chest is expanding more easily!
- Feel how your back is arching and rounding more easily!
- Feel the improvement!

feel the difference!

let your body move freely

12

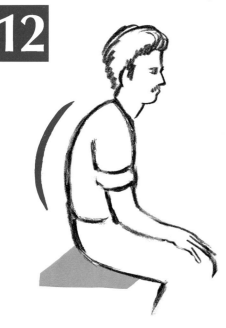

Sit back in your chair and let your back become rounded or "slumped."

- Notice that your chest becomes flattened and your breathing becomes restricted.
- Notice that the muscles of your neck and back are strained, and the flexibility of your neck is limited.

13

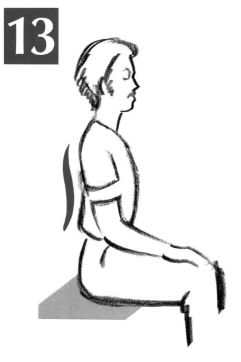

Now sit on the forward edge of your chair, with your lower back slightly arched and your weight supported by your pelvic sitting bones.

- Notice that your neck and shoulders are relaxed and free to move, and your stomach muscles are relaxed.
- Notice that your chest is expanding easily.
- Feel the difference in your breathing!

You have completed **"Full Breathing."** When you stand up and walk around, feel how relaxed your entire body is and feel the improvement in your posture!

Enjoy your improvement!

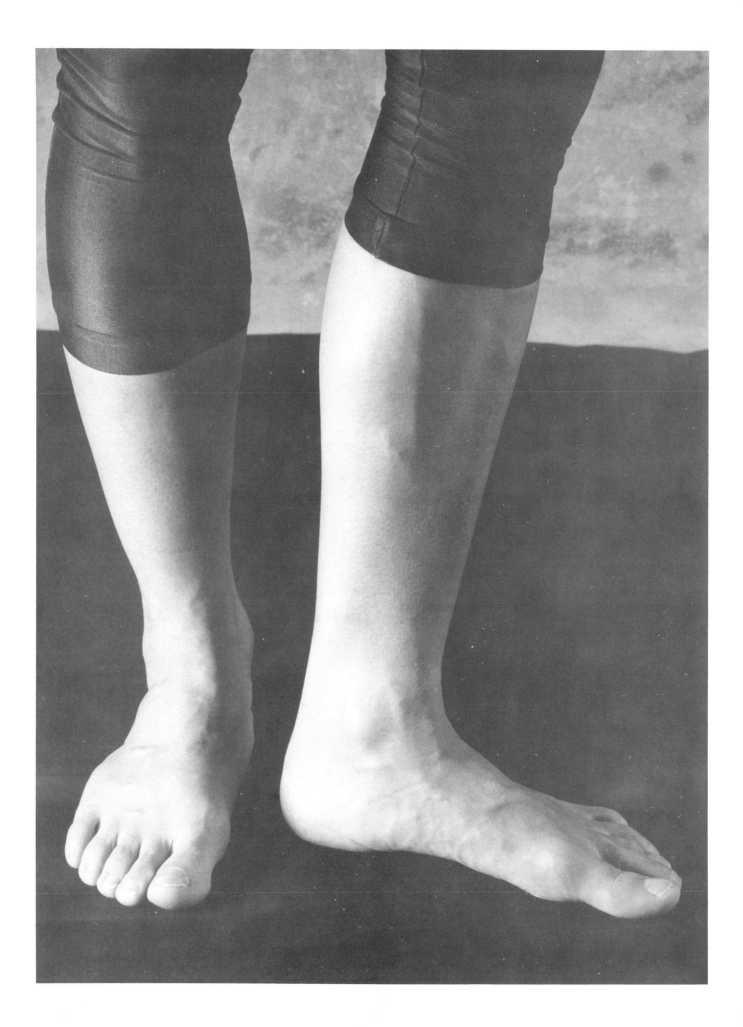

8 FLEXIBLE FEET

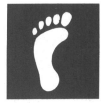

Langston J., fifty-two, had been a mail-carrier for over fifteen years. In spite of being physically active, his feet, legs, and back ached daily, his posture had become hunched over, and his body was visibly tilted to the right. We gave Langston the basic Relaxercise program. Within a few weeks, his posture was more upright and symmetrical, and he had gained significant relief from his muscular discomfort.

If our bodies had been designed to stand still we would probably not have feet. We would more likely have a wide, solid base of support, like the base of a statue. But our bodies are marvelously designed for movement and instead of having a wide, solid base of support, we have feet. It is the narrowness and flexibility of our feet that makes movement so easy. Made up of twenty-six small, movable bones, our feet efficiently support the weight of our entire body.

Thousands of years ago, our ancestors walked much more than we do today, and they walked on a much greater variety of surfaces: shifting sand, rocky slopes, sun-baked earth, and so on. Their feet had to be strong and flexible in order to adjust to the different surfaces beneath them. But today, most of us live in cities and use our feet in very limited ways. When we walk, the surface beneath us is almost always flat, hard, and unyielding. We choose our shoes to match our clothing instead of provide us with maximum stability and flexibility. Slowly but surely, our feet lose some of their natural agility. They become stiff and support our body's weight less efficiently. This inevitably has an adverse effect on our posture.

"Flexible Feet" will help restore the natural flexibility of your feet. Your posture will improve and your stability will increase, so that every movement you make can be freer and easier.

FLEXIBLE FEET

You will need a hard or firmly cushioned chair or seat.

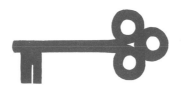

Use the Relaxercise Keys

- **Go slowly.**

- **Make each movement small and easy.**

- **Relax as much as you can.**

- **Rest briefly after each movement.**

STARTING POSITION
You can do this exercise while wearing
shoes, but for maximum effectiveness,
remove your shoes before you begin.
Sit on the forward part of your chair or seat
and rest your hands on your thighs.
Rest your feet flat on the floor, shoulder
width apart, directly below your knees.

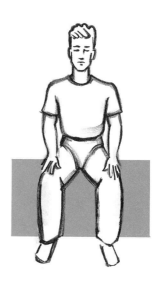

1

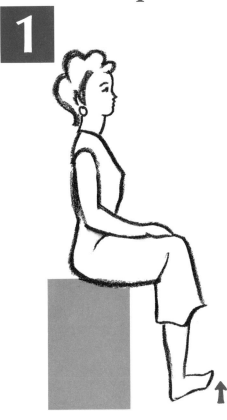

Very slowly lift the forward part (the toes and ball) of your right foot slightly. Then return to the starting position and rest.

- Keep your heel on the floor.
- Don't stretch. Lift the forward part of your right foot **very** slightly.
- Relax your right foot and leg as much as possible.
- As you lift the forward part of your foot, feel the slight movement in your right knee and hip joint.
- Breathe freely.

2

Very slowly lift your right heel slightly. Then return to the starting position and rest.

- Keep the forward part of your foot on the floor.
- Use as little muscular effort as possible.
- Make each movement small and easy.
- As you lift your heel, notice whether the pressure moves more toward your big toe or your little toe. Try to spread the weight evenly.
- Notice how the movement in your ankle affects your knee, leg, and lower back.

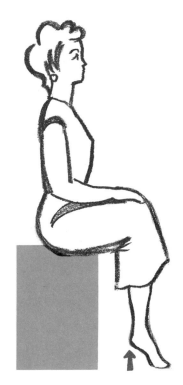

pause to rest after each movement

3

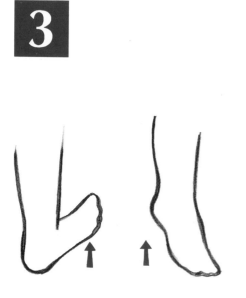

Alternately: lift the forward part of your right foot slightly; then return to the starting position, and relax. Then, lift your heel slightly—and then return to the starting position and relax.

- Go slowly. Make each movement smooth and relaxed.
- Relax your back and chest.
- Feel the slight movement in your right knee and right hip.
- When you lift your heel, your pelvis may tilt forward slightly, and when you lift the forward part of your foot, your pelvis may tilt back slightly.

And now, rest for a moment.

- Feel how your right foot is resting in closer contact with the floor.
- Does your right foot feel more relaxed than your left foot?

4

Very slowly lift the forward part of your left foot slightly. Then return to the starting position and rest.

- Keep your heel on the floor.
- Relax your left foot and leg as much as you can.
- Feel the slight movement in your left knee and hip joint.

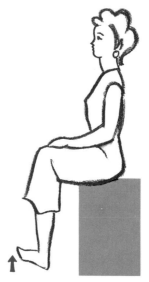

don't stretch or strain

5 Very slowly lift your left heel slightly. Then return to the starting position and rest.

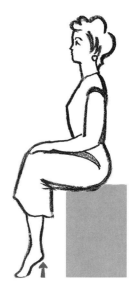

- Keep the forward part of your foot on the floor.
- Relax your left leg.
- Do not strain your foot or ankle.
- Notice whether more pressure moves toward your little toe or your big toe. Try to spread the weight evenly.
- Feel how the movement in your ankle affects your knee, leg, and lower back.

6 First lift the forward part of your left foot slightly, then return to the starting position and rest. Next, lift your left heel slightly, and return to the starting position and rest.

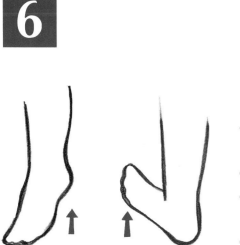

- Go slowly. Make the movement smooth and continuous.
- Relax your back and chest.
- Feel the slight movement in your left knee and hip.
- When you lift your heel, your pelvis tilts forward slightly. When you lift the forward part of your foot, your pelvis tilts back slightly.

Rest for a moment.

- Is your left foot resting in closer contact with the floor?
- Does your left foot feel more relaxed?

feel the difference! and then continue . . .

7

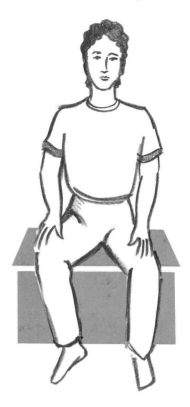

Slowly lift the inside edge of your right foot slightly. Then return to the starting position and rest.

- Relax your toes, ankle, and leg.
- To make it easier, lift the weight of your left buttock slightly, while lifting the inside edge of your right foot. As you lift the weight of your left buttock very slightly, your weight will shift toward your right buttock.
- Feel your foot's weight roll to the outside edge.

8

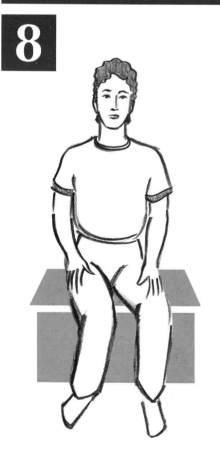

Slowly lift the outside edge of your right foot slightly. Then return to the starting position and rest.

- Relax your left foot and leg.
- Feel your foot's weight roll to the inside edge.
- Notice how your right knee moves a little to the left.
- To make the movement easier, lift the weight of your right buttock slightly, while lifting the outside edge of your right foot. As you lift the weight very slightly your weight will shift toward your left buttock.

relax after each movement

9

Alternately lift the inside edge of your right foot slightly so your foot's weight rolls to the outside edge. Then return to the starting position, and lift the outside edge of your right foot slightly so your foot's weight rolls to the inside edge.

- Relax your right foot and leg as much as possible.
- Breathe freely, so your chest and spine can move easily.
- Notice that your right knee moves to the right and left a little.
- Notice that your pelvis shifts right and left a little.
- Keep your knee still and see what happens. Is the movement easier or more difficult?

10

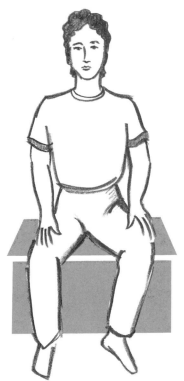

Very slowly lift the inside edge of your left foot slightly. Then return to the starting position and rest.

- Feel the weight of your foot roll to the outside edge.
- Relax your foot, toes, ankle, and entire leg.
- Notice that your left knee and thigh move to the left slightly.
- To make it easier, lift the weight of your right buttock slightly, while lifting the inside edge of your left foot. As you lift the weight of your right buttock your weight will roll toward your left buttock.

exhale with each movement

relax your leg, ankle, foot, and toes

11

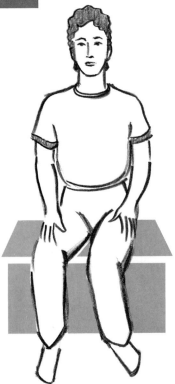

Slowly lift the outside edge of your left foot very slightly. Then return to the starting position and rest.

- Feel the weight of your foot roll toward the inside edge.
- Notice your left knee moving to the right slightly.
- To make the movement easier, lift the weight of your left buttock slightly, while raising the outside edge of your left foot. When you lift the weight of your left buttock a little, your weight will roll toward your right buttock.

12

Alternately lift the inside edge of your left foot slightly so your foot's weight rolls to the outside edge. Then return to the starting position and lift the outside edge of your left foot slightly so your foot's weight rolls to the inside edge.

- Go easily. Don't stretch or strain your foot.
- As you alternate, your left knee and your pelvis move a little, from side to side.
- Keep your knee still and see what happens. Is the movement easier or more difficult?

repeat each movement 4 to 8 times

And now, rest for a moment.

- Feel how relaxed your feet are!
- Feel how comfortably they are resting on the floor.

13

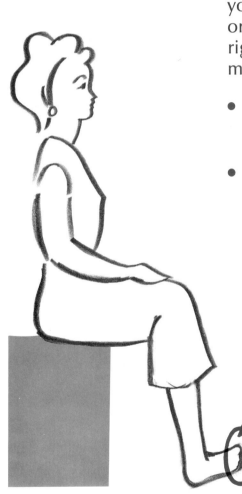

Move your right foot forward on the floor 4 to 6 inches. Then lift the forward part of your right foot very slightly. Keep your heel on the floor. Rotate the forward part of your right foot slowly in a clockwise circular movement.

- Imagine your big toe is moving the hand of a clock around its dial, very slowly.
- Feel the slight circular movement in your right hip joint, pelvis, and lower back. Let your whole body—your back, neck, chest, and shoulders—join the circular movement.

rest whenever you like

rotate slowly 4 to 8 times

14

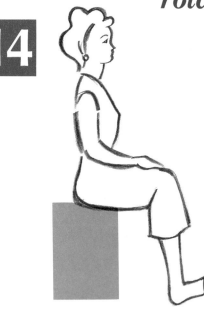

Now, change direction: Lift the forward part of your right foot very slightly. Keep your heel on the floor. Rotate the forward part of your right foot, slowly, in a counterclockwise circle.

- Relax your entire body.
- Notice that the slight circular movement in your right hip joint, lower back, and pelvis has changed direction.

And now, rest.

- Feel the difference in your right foot!

15

Move your left foot forward on the floor 4 to 6 inches. Then lift the forward part of your left foot very slightly. Keep your heel on the floor. Rotate the forward part of your left foot, slowly, in a clockwise circular movement.

- Imagine your big toe is moving the hand of a clock around its dial.
- Relax your leg, ankle, foot, and toes as much as possible.
- Feel the slight circular movement in your left hip joint, pelvis, and back.
- Let your whole body—your back, neck, chest, and shoulders—join the circular movement.

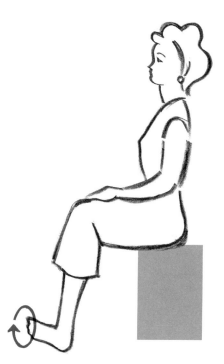

stop to rest whenever you like

Now change direction: Lift the forward part of your left foot very slightly. Keep your heel on the floor. Rotate the forward part of your left foot, slowly, in a counterclockwise circle.

- Notice that the slight circular movement in your left hip joint, lower back, and pelvis has changed direction.

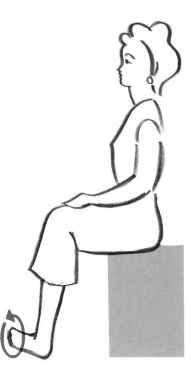

 And now, rest.

Feel the improved contact between your feet and the floor. Feel how relaxed your entire body is!

You have completed **"Flexible Feet."** When you stand up and walk around, notice how relaxed and balanced your feet, legs, and hips are. Feel how securely your feet are supporting you.

Enjoy the improvement!

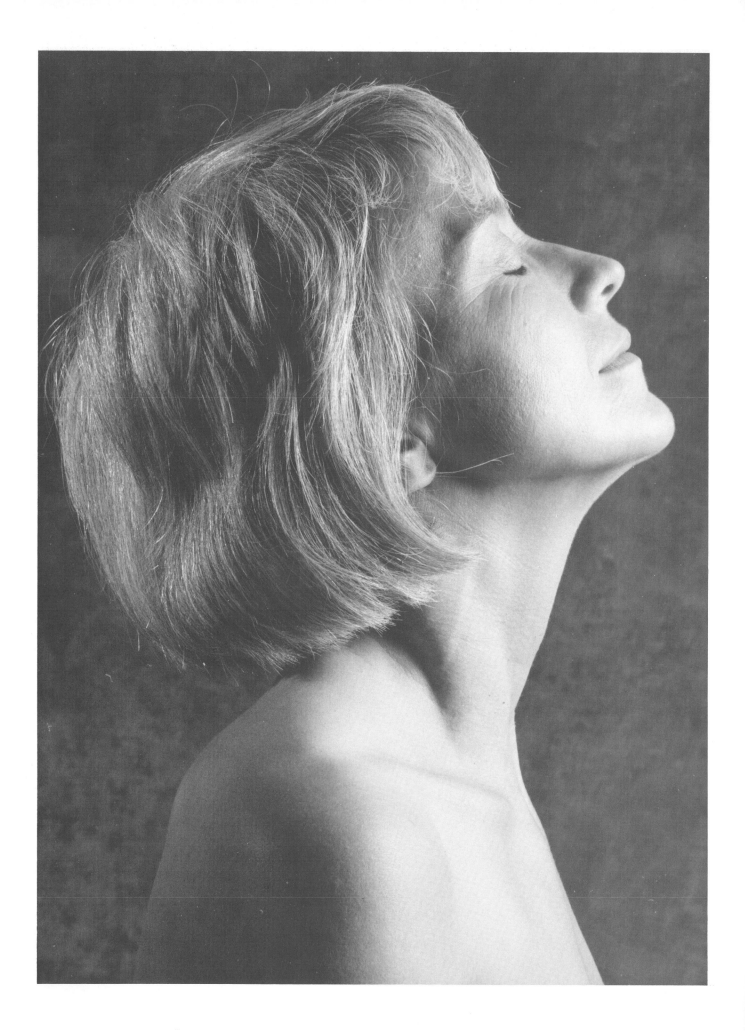

9 FACE & JAW TREATMENT

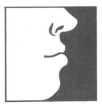

Diana J., thirty-one, suffered chronic jaw pain and tension for over seven years. It began as unconscious nighttime teeth grinding and eventually became a constant discomfort, often accompanied by headaches and neck pain. When Diana came to us, she had tried just about everything her dentist had to offer, but to no avail. By using Relaxercise, she quickly changed the muscular habit patterns responsible for her pain and gained the comfort and relief she had been wanting for so long.

Jaw and facial tension is a very common stress-related problem. The most easily recognized symptoms are unconscious grinding or clenching of the teeth, pain around the eyes, headaches, and neck pain. Recent evidence suggests that chronic jaw tension can even cause shoulder pain and lower back problems.

Jaw tension also makes your face appear tight and drawn and contributes to the development of unwanted lines and wrinkles. One of the most effective things you can do to ensure that your face stays youthful and attractive is to keep it relaxed and free of tension.

"Face and Jaw Treatment" will give you powerful and effective techniques for relaxing your jaw and facial muscles. It will dissolve habitual patterns of muscular tension and balance your facial muscle tone. As tension disappears, your face will look and feel relaxed and youthful.

FACE AND JAW TREATMENT

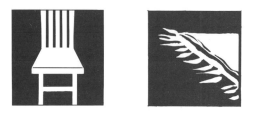

You will need a comfortable chair or seat, or an exercise mat or rug.

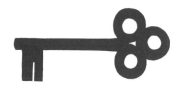

Use the Relaxercise Keys

- **Go slowly.**

- **Make each movement small and easy.**

- **Relax as much as you can.**

- **Rest briefly after each movement.**

STARTING POSITIONS

Seated Sit in a comfortable chair or seat. Rest your hands on your thighs. Rest your feet flat on the floor, shoulder width apart, directly below your knees.

Lying down Lie on your back and rest your arms by your sides. Either stretch out your legs, or bend your knees, and rest your feet flat on the floor, shoulder width apart, directly below your knees.

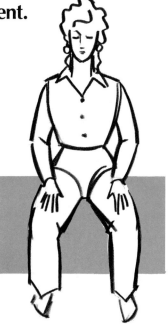

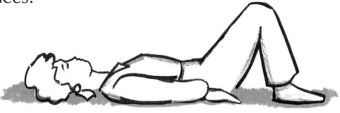

1

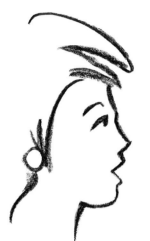

Very slowly open and close your mouth a little bit.

- Relax your face, neck, throat, and tongue.
- When you open your mouth, does your lower jaw move straight down or does it veer slightly to the right or left?
- Notice that your head moves back slightly as you open your mouth.

2

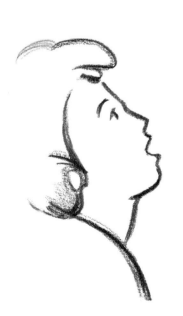

Simultaneously, open your mouth while tilting your head back a little. Then slowly close your mouth and bring your head back to the starting position.

- Notice that tilting your head back helps your mouth to open more easily.
- To make this movement easier, relax your neck.

pause to rest after each movement

3

Open your mouth a little and keep it open. Slowly move your lower jaw to the right **very slightly**. Then let your jaw return to the middle, close your mouth, and rest.

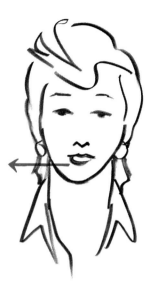

- Put your left forefinger on your chin so you can feel the movement of your lower jaw more clearly. Does your lower jaw move smoothly or does its movement seem rough and uneven at certain points?
- Go slowly and relax your jaw, so the movement can be smooth and easy.

And now, rest.

- Feel the right side of your mouth and jaw beginning to relax!

4

Open your mouth a little and keep it open. Slowly move your lower jaw **very slightly** to the left. Then let your jaw return to the middle, close your mouth, and rest.

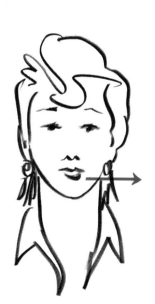

- Put your left forefinger on your chin so you can feel the movement of your jaw more clearly.
- Does moving your jaw to the left feel different from moving it to the right?
- To make this movement smooth and comfortable, go slowly and move your jaw only a small amount.

relax your jaw, neck, and shoulders

make each movement relaxed and easy

Rest for a moment.

- Feel your jaw, mouth, and entire face relaxing. As your jaw relaxes, headaches, neck, and shoulder pain often begin to disappear.

5

Open your mouth a little and keep it open. Alternately, slowly move your lower jaw to the left a little and then to the right a little. Move your lower jaw slowly from side to side.

- Use as **little** muscular effort as possible.
- Relax your eyes. Notice how they are moving from side to side slightly.
- Rest often so the muscles of your face and jaw do not get tired.

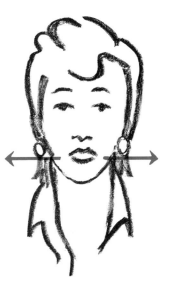

6

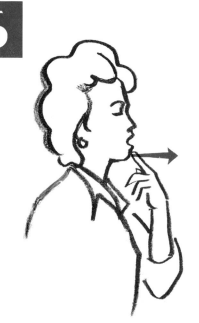

Open your mouth a little and keep it open. Slowly move your lower jaw forward a little so your lower teeth are slightly more forward than your upper teeth. Then let your jaw return to its normal position and rest.

- Put a finger on your chin so you can feel the movement more clearly. When your jaw moves forward, does it move straight forward, or does it veer slightly to the right or left?

go slowly and rest after each movement

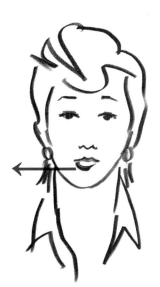

Open your mouth a little, move your lower jaw forward, and keep it there. Slowly move your jaw to the right a little. Then let your jaw return to the middle and rest.

- Relax your tongue and throat as much as possible.
- Breathe freely.

Open your mouth, move your lower jaw forward, and keep it there. Slowly move your lower jaw a little to the left. Then let your lower jaw return to the middle and rest.

- Relax your arms, stomach, and legs.
- Does moving your jaw to the left feel different than moving it to the right?

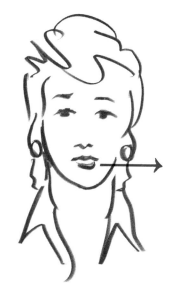

make each movement slow, easy and comfortable

use as little effort as possible

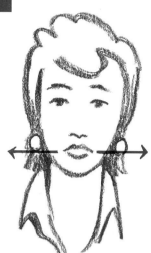

Open your mouth a little, move your lower jaw forward, and keep it there. Then alternately, move your lower jaw slowly to the right a little and then to the left a little. Move your lower jaw from side to side, gently.

- Make this movement smooth and continuous.
- Relax your face and entire body as much as you can.
- Don't let your jaw get tired.

Rest for a moment.

- Feel the ease and relaxation in your face and neck.
- Notice how relaxed and comfortable your mouth and jaw feel.

Measure your improvement: Simply open and close your mouth a few times.

- Let gravity and the weight of your lower jaw open your mouth gently.
- Notice that when your mouth and jaw are closed and relaxed, there is a slight space between your upper and lower teeth.
- Notice how much more easily and comfortably your mouth can open now.

You have completed **"Face and Jaw Treatment."** When you stand up and walk around, feel the relaxation in your face, jaw, and entire body.

Enjoy your improvement!

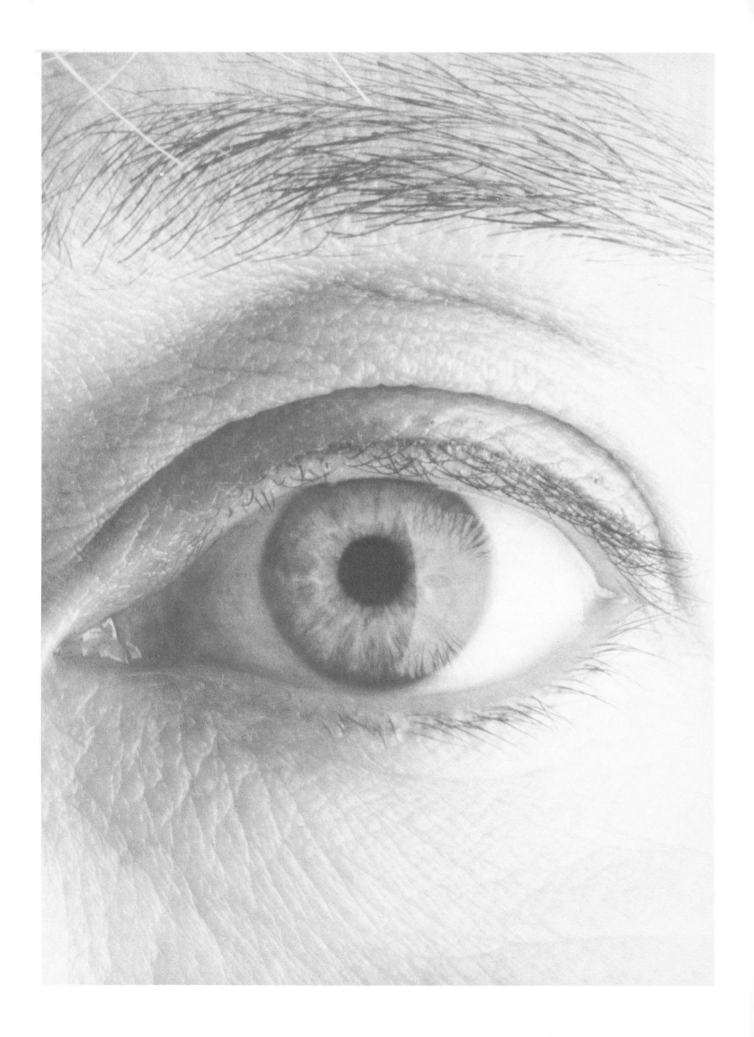

10 RELAXED EYESIGHT

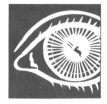

Joanne P., a twenty-seven-year-old executive secretary in a multi-national corporation, sat at a desk answering phone calls and typing reports for eight to ten hours each day. Referred to us by her physical therapist, she complained of headaches, eyestrain, and shoulder and back pain. Relaxercise exercises helped Joanne to change the way she used her body while working. As she learned to relax her eyesight and improve her sitting posture, Joanne's symptoms began to disappear.

We depend on sight more than any other sense to supply us with information about the world around us. In order to maintain healthy eyesight, our eyes need to use their entire range of vision, from close up to far in the distance. But in today's world, we spend most of our time focusing on objects close to us. For example, we use *near vision* while reading, watching television, scanning computer monitors, and working with machines. The predominant use of near vision is one of the primary causes of chronic eyestrain and of tension in the neck, shoulders, and back.

Seeing involves an intricate coordination between your eyes, brain, and body. This unique exercise will help you to use your eyes in a more relaxed way. Your quality of vision will improve, and you will learn how to reduce eyestrain. Because there is a close neuromuscular relationship between your eyes and the rest of your body, you will find that as your vision becomes more relaxed, tension will disappear from your face, neck, and shoulders.

RELAXED EYESIGHT

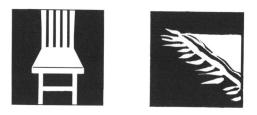

You will need either a comfortable chair or seat, or an exercise mat or rug.

Use the Relaxercise Keys

- **Go slowly.**

- **Make each movement small and easy.**

- **Relax as much as you can.**

- **Rest briefly after each movement.**

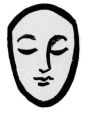

THERE ARE TWO WAYS TO DO THIS EXERCISE:
1. Read each movement instruction and then close your eyes while doing the movement.
2. Have a friend read the exercise aloud.

Note: If you wear contact lenses or glasses, remove them before you begin.

STARTING POSITIONS

Seated Sit on a comfortable chair or seat. Rest your hands on your thighs. Rest your feet flat on the floor, shoulder width apart, directly below your knees.

Lying down Lie flat on your back and rest your arms alongside your body. Either stretch out your legs, or bend your knees and place your feet flat on the floor, shoulder width apart, directly below your knees.

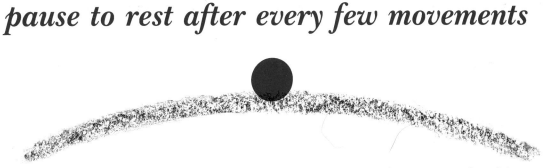

Close your eyes. In your imagination, pretend you are looking at a round ball which is sitting on a distant horizon line straight ahead. In your imagination, choose the ball's color and size.

Imagine the ball moving very slowly to the right a little and then to the left a little along the distant horizon. Close your eyes and move them slowly from side to side, as you follow the ball in your imagination.

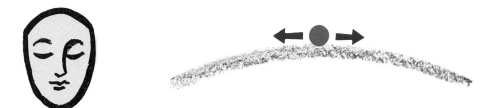

- Don't strain your eyes.
- Move your eyes very slowly.
- Make each movement small and easy.
- Breathe freely.
- Your eyes will probably move unevenly at some points. The ball may seem to skip suddenly, or you may lose sight of the ball from time to time.

repeat each movement 4 to 8 times

2

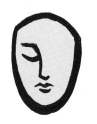

Now pay attention to your right eye only. Imagine the ball moving slowly a little to the right, and then back to the middle, along the distant horizon line. Close your eyes and, in your imagination, let your right eye follow the ball.

- Pay attention to your right eye only.
- Make the movement small, relaxed, and comfortable.
- Do not strain your right eye by looking too far to the right.
- If the movement of your right eye is uneven at some points, slow down.
- Relax your face, neck, and shoulders.

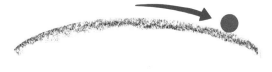

3

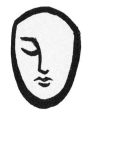

Pay attention to your right eye only. Imagine the ball moving slowly a little to the left, and then back to the middle, along the distant horizon. Close your eyes and follow the ball with your right eye.

- Use as little effort as possible.
- Do your eyes seem to lose sight of the ball, or does the ball skip at some points? To make the ball move smoothly, go more slowly.

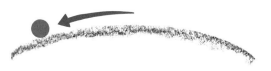

breathe freely

Rest and relax your eyes.

- Feel the difference between your right eye and your left eye!

4

Pay attention to your left eye only. Imagine the ball moving slowly a little to the left, and then back to the middle, along the distant horizon. Close your eyes and follow the ball with your left eye.

- Make this a slight, comfortable movement.
- Relax your jaw and forehead.
- Don't strain your left eye. The movement will improve automatically.

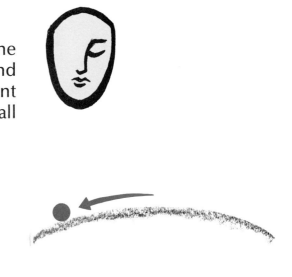

5

Pay attention to your left eye only. Imagine the ball moving slowly a little to the right, and then back to the middle, along the distant horizon. Close your eyes and follow the ball with your left eye.

- Go very slowly.
- Relax your left eye as much as possible.

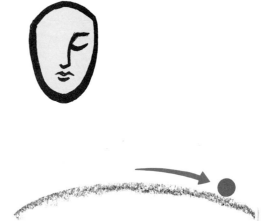

relax your eyes and take your time

use as little muscular effort as possible

Imagine the ball moving slowly to the left a little, and then to the right a little, along the distant horizon. Close your eyes and follow the ball with both eyes.

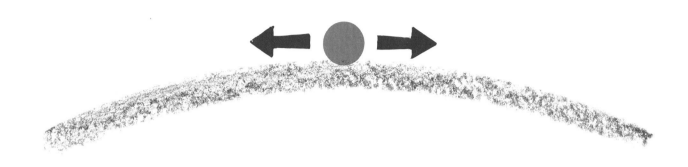

- Are your eyes moving more smoothly now?

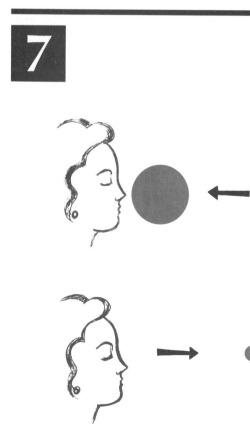

7

Imagine that the ball and horizon are very far away. Follow the ball in your imagination as it begins to move slowly closer and closer, gradually getting larger, until it stops just a few feet away from your face. Then imagine the ball going away again, slowly getting smaller and smaller as it returns to the distant horizon. Pause to rest when the ball reaches the horizon.

- Notice how at some distances, it is easy to imagine the ball clearly, but at other distances, the ball appears to jump or go out of focus. Going slowly will help the ball stay in focus.

pause to rest after every few movements

8 Imagine the ball moving along the horizon to the right, and then imagine it stopping at the far right side. Then follow the ball in your imagination as it slowly comes closer and closer, getting larger and larger, until it softly touches the right side of your face. Then imagine the ball slowly becoming smaller as it returns to the far right side of the distant horizon.

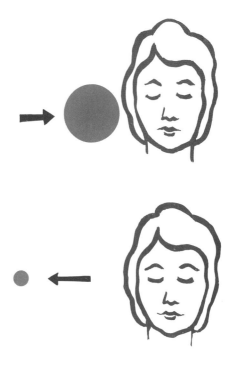

- Don't strain your eyes. Make the movement relaxed and easy.
- Use as little effort as possible.
- Imagine the ball stopping at various points along the way so you can develop a clearer focus.

9

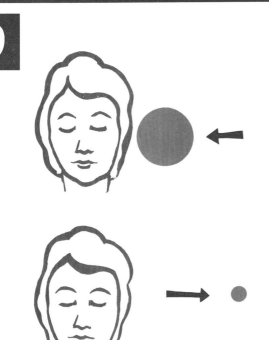

Imagine the ball moving along the distant horizon to the left. Imagine the ball stopping on the far left side of the horizon. Then watch the ball in your imagination as it slowly comes closer and closer, getting larger and larger, until it softly touches the left side of your face. Then imagine the ball slowly becoming smaller as it returns to the left side of the distant horizon.

- Relax your eyes, face, neck, and shoulders as much as possible.
- Imagine the ball stopping at various points along the way so you can develop a clearer focus.

feel the difference! and then continue . . .

relax your entire body as much as possible

10

With your eyes closed, slowly look to the right and to the left a few times.

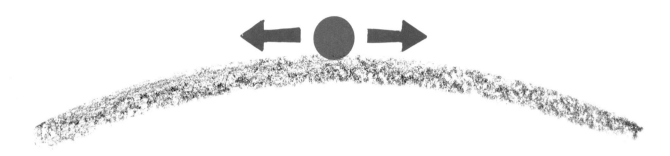

- Notice that the movement of your eyes has become much smoother and easier!
- Notice how much farther to the right and left you can move your eyes without strain.

And now, open your eyes.

- Notice how your eyes feel calm and rested.
- Notice how clear your vision is.
- Notice that your face and neck feel more relaxed, too!

You have completed **"Relaxed Eyesight."** When you stand up and walk around, feel the relaxation of your entire body.

Enjoy the improvement!

EYE CARE TIPS

The following suggestions can help you maintain healthy, relaxed vision:

- Use your eyes' full range of motion: left, right, up, down, near and far.

- If your work involves the use of near vision, periodically rest your eyes by closing them for at *least* a moment or two every hour.

- When you need to use near vision for long periods of time, shift your gaze out a window or around the room every so often.

- Your office or work area should be well lit, without glare or shadows.

- When working at a desk, try using a book or copy holder to reduce the tendency to lean forward while reading.

- If your work involves the use of a computer video display terminal (VDT), read the VDT eye care information in the "Ergonomic Tips" chapter.

- Practice relaxed eyesight by eliminating unnecessary muscular effort and tension from your vision.

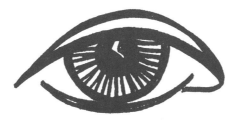

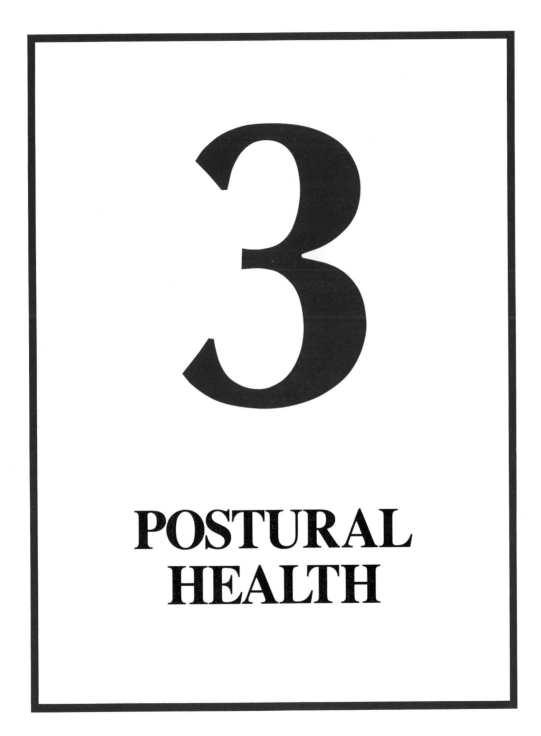

3

POSTURAL
HEALTH

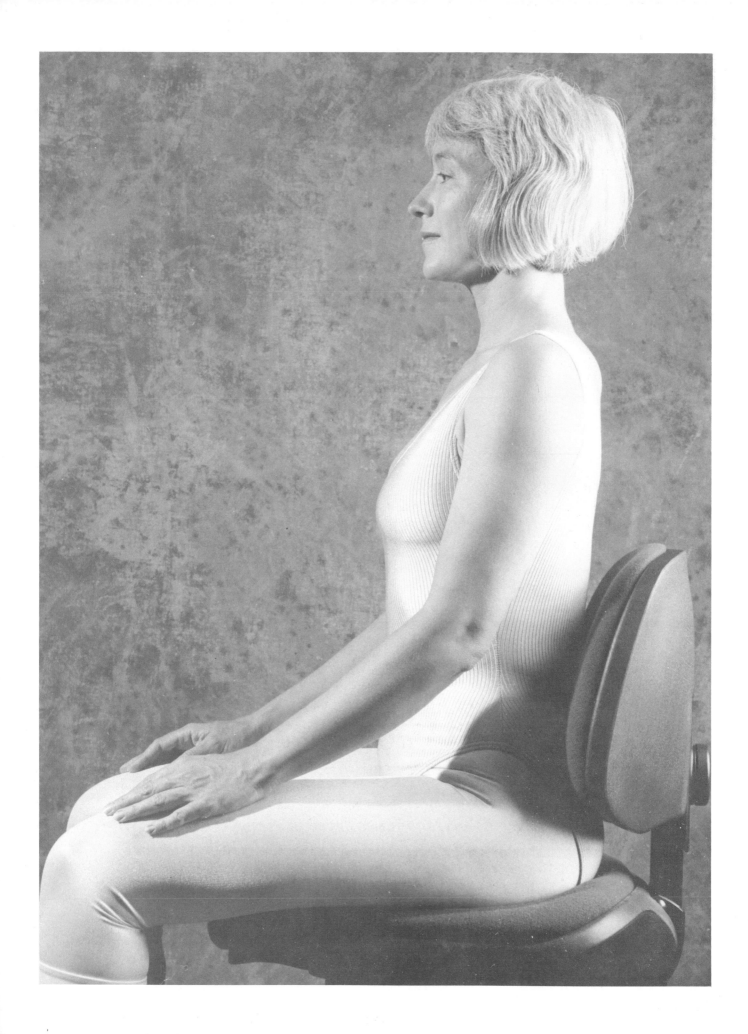

THE ART OF DYNAMIC SITTING

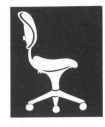

Marilyn S., a twenty-six-year-old semiconductor worker, came to see us after her employer heard about our exercises for office workers. She had been a healthy, pain-free person until she began sitting eight hours a day at work. Now she suffered neck, shoulder, and back pain almost every day. We gave Marilyn some Relaxercise exercises to use at home and work and taught her how to use the principles of "Dynamic Sitting." In just a few days she was pain free.

Never before have men and women spent so much time sitting. We live and work in a world in which most of us sit in a chair or seat from eight to fifteen hours a day! From kitchen table to car, from office to movie theater, from chair to sofa, we spend our day moving from one seated position to another.

Sitting for long periods of time is muscularly stressful for your body. Though sitting may take the weight off your feet, it actually increases the stress on your back. In fact, the pressure on your spine can be as much as 50 percent more when sitting than when standing.

If you sit for more than four hours per day, your *sitting posture* may be affecting the health and comfort of your neck, shoulders, and back. If you frequently experience aches or stiffness in your neck, shoulders, or back, your sitting posture is probably at the root of the problem. If your occupation requires you to sit in a chair, we advise that you take the time to develop a safe and healthy sitting posture.

This chapter introduces Dynamic Sitting, the healthiest way to sit. Dynamic Sitting is **not** a static position. With Dynamic Sitting, your body is seated but not fixed, constrained, or restricted, and your muscles are neither strained nor overworked. When you use the principles of Dynamic Sitting, you can move freely, bend and shift your weight easily and efficiently, and maintain a healthy back and neck, even while sitting for long periods of time.

THE ELEMENTS OF DYNAMIC SITTING

USING YOUR SKELETAL SUPPORT

Nature designed your skeleton to support your body and hold it upright, counteracting the powerful downward pull of gravity. When your skeleton is properly aligned, your bones can withstand more pressure than steel.

Poor sitting posture **prevents** your skeleton from providing your body with efficient structural support. With poor sitting posture, muscular discomfort quickly develops, because your muscles and ligaments are working overtime in order to hold your body upright. When your muscles and ligaments are doing the work that your skeleton should be doing, they become tense, over-used, and strained. Even if your muscles are large and strong, your bones are capable of supporting your body's weight with far greater efficiency.

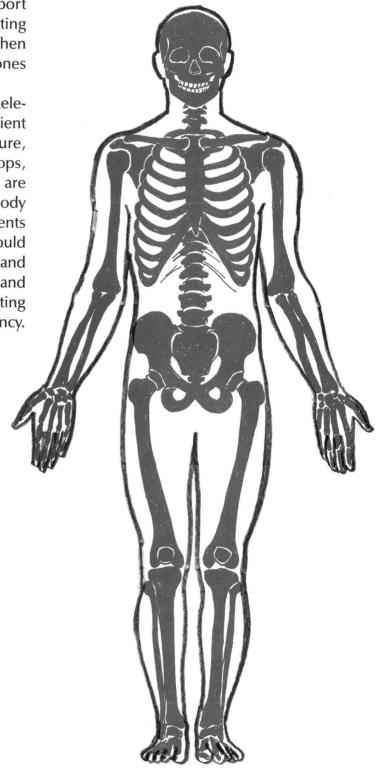

YOUR PELVIS

When you sit, your pelvis becomes your body's main source of structural support. Your pelvis is able to support your body's weight easily and efficiently. But if you sit with your back and neck rounded, much of your body's weight is thrown backward so that your body loses the support provided by your pelvis. Without the structural support of your pelvis, tremendous pressure and strain is placed on your muscles, ligaments, and spinal discs. This is why habitual rounding of the lower back is the most common cause of chronic back, neck, and shoulder discomfort.

Your pelvis supports your body effectively only when your lower back is slightly arched. With your back arched slightly, your weight is efficiently supported by your **pelvic sitting bones**, the two bony projections of your pelvis. They have a rounded shape on which your body's weight can balance. When your weight is efficiently supported by your sitting bones, your back is most relaxed and flexible—able to tilt, bend, and turn with hardly any muscular effort at all.

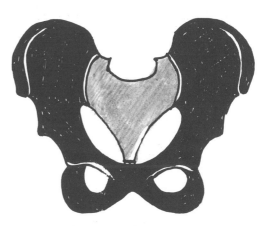

Pelvic 'sitting bones'

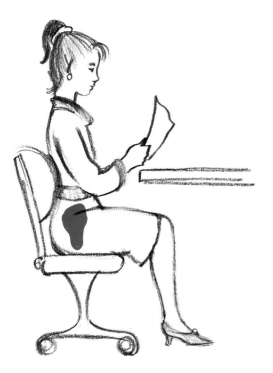

Sitting with pelvic support

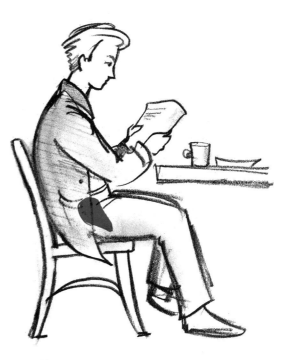

Sitting without pelvic support

BALANCE

It is important to distribute the weight of your body equally over both your pelvic sitting bones. We frequently develop a habit of leaning to one side much more than to the other. This overworks the muscles on one side of your back and neck and, over time, can distort the shape of your spine. When one side of your pelvis chronically supports more of your weight, problems such as scoliosis (an S-shaped curvature of the spine) can develop in your lower back.

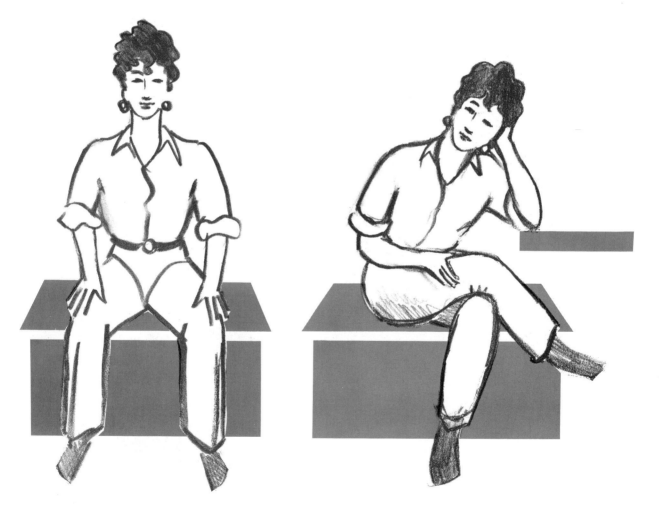

Good sitting posture   **Poor sitting posture**

YOUR CHAIR

Unfortunately, most conventional chairs are poorly designed. They lack adequate support for your lower back and cannot be adjusted to fit either your individual physical structure or sitting needs. Usually, when you lean back or sit toward the rear of most conventional chairs, your back becomes rounded and your lumbar arch disappears. For information on well-designed chairs, see the "Ergonomic Tips" chapter and the "Resource Directory."

Dynamic Sitting posture is easier to maintain when you sit on the forward edge of your chair or seat. When you sit on the forward edge of your seat, your lower back tends to arch naturally, and your pelvic sitting bones can support you, no matter what kind of chair you are sitting on.

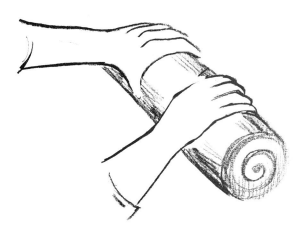

When you sit or lean back in your chair, we recommend that you try using a low back support or roll. You can buy a low back roll from an orthopedic or back care supply store, or you can easily make one yourself.

To make a low back support:
Roll a small towel into a tight cylindrical shape with a diameter of one to four inches. Place the rolled-up towel between your lower back and the back of your chair. This will effectively help you maintain the arch of your lower back. Find the diameter most comfortable for your back. Every so often, vary the diameter; this will help maintain the flexibility of your back. Low back strain can often be reduced instantly by using this simple technique.

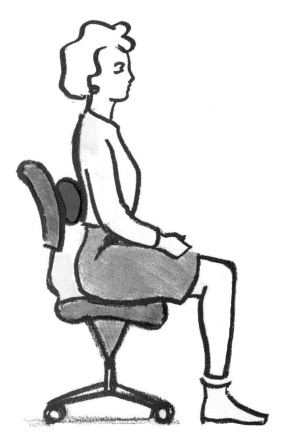

YOUR NECK AND SHOULDERS

Many people think that tucking your chin in is part of good posture. This idea originated with the classic military posture and is actually a dangerous misconception. When your chin is tucked in, your neck muscles become overstretched, the curve of your upper spine is diminished, and the movement of your head and neck is severely restricted. To maintain the comfort of your neck, your head should be supported by your spine, and **not** by the muscles of your neck. Hold your head comfortably upright, not too far back and not tilted up or down too far. Held upright comfortably, your neck muscles can be relaxed and your head can move freely, without strain.

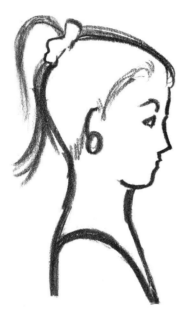

When sitting at a table or desk, we tend to lean forward with our head and neck. This invariably makes our neck and shoulders tense, because the muscles of our neck and upper back are overworked and strained. You can protect your neck and shoulders by sitting closer to your work surface. Sit on the forward edge of your chair or as close as possible to your desk or table. Then, **lean forward from your hip joints** rather than by rounding your back. You can also reduce the need to lean forward by tilting the angle of either your work surface or work materials. Adjustable work surfaces and book and paper holders are available.

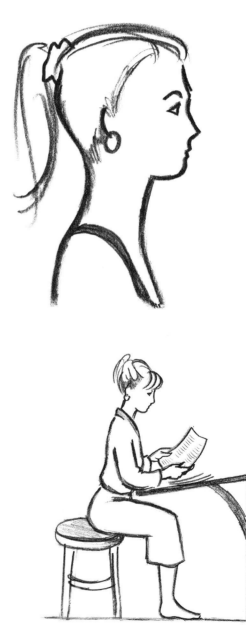

YOUR LEGS AND FEET

Your legs and feet play an important role in healthy sitting posture. Dynamic Sitting is easiest and most natural when your feet are resting flat on the floor, about shoulder width apart, directly below your knees. In this position, your legs and feet are free of tension, your hip joints are more flexible, and your lower back is more relaxed. Your feet should be able to move freely as you shift your weight, bend, or turn, while sitting. If your feet do not reach the floor, it is a good idea to use a footrest.

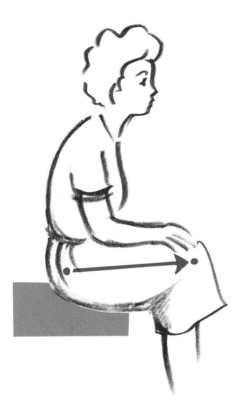 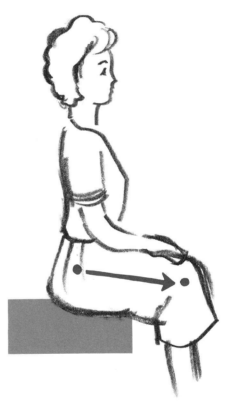

When your knees are higher than the level of your hips, your lower back tends to round. Keeping your knees slightly below the level of your hips will help you maintain the arch of your lower back. Avoid sitting with your knees close together. This creates tension in your legs, pelvis, and stomach.

Whenever possible, avoid crossing your legs or ankles while sitting. Crossing your legs or ankles puts more of your weight on one of your pelvic sitting bones. When this happens, your spine curves, your lower back rounds, and the alignment of your entire body becomes unbalanced.

CONCLUSION

The secret of Dynamic Sitting is to utilize full skeletal support so your body is free to move easily and comfortably while you sit.

By using the principles of Dynamic Sitting, you can strengthen your back, prevent back pain, and gain tremendous relief from the muscular stress caused by poor and restrictive sitting habits. The fatigue usually experienced after many hours of sitting will disappear. As your muscles relax, you will find yourself feeling more comfortable and energetic.

Dynamic Sitting can make a profound difference in your daily life. Try it! Though it may feel unusual and unfamiliar at first, after a while it will begin to be a comfortable, healthy habit. Then you can say good-bye to all those aches and pains associated with long periods of sitting.

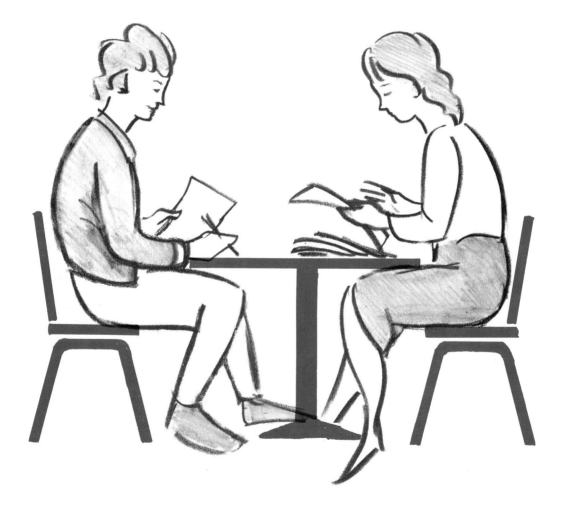

Poor sitting posture = Back pain

DYNAMIC SITTING CHECKLIST

- If possible, use an adjustable ergonomic chair. If you use a conventional chair, try sitting on the forward edge of the seat.
- If you lean back in your chair, make sure your lower back is supported by a contoured seat back or a lumbar roll.
- Balance your weight evenly on both pelvic sitting bones.

- Arch your lower back slightly.
- Arch your neck slightly.
- Relax your shoulders.
- Relax your abdomen.
- Rest both your feet flat on the floor.
- Breathe freely and easily.
- Change your sitting position frequently.
- Let go of unnecessary muscular effort and tension in your body.

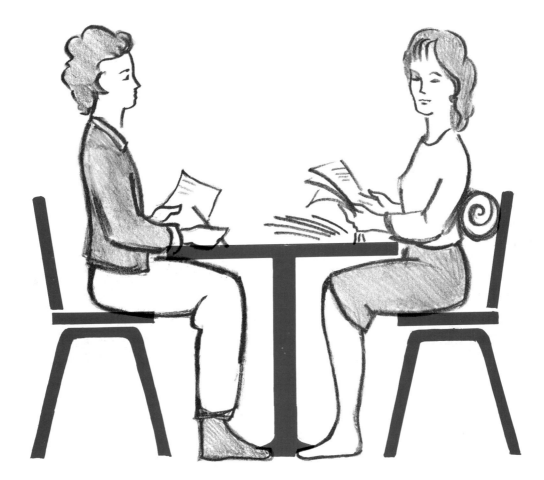

Dynamic sitting = Comfort

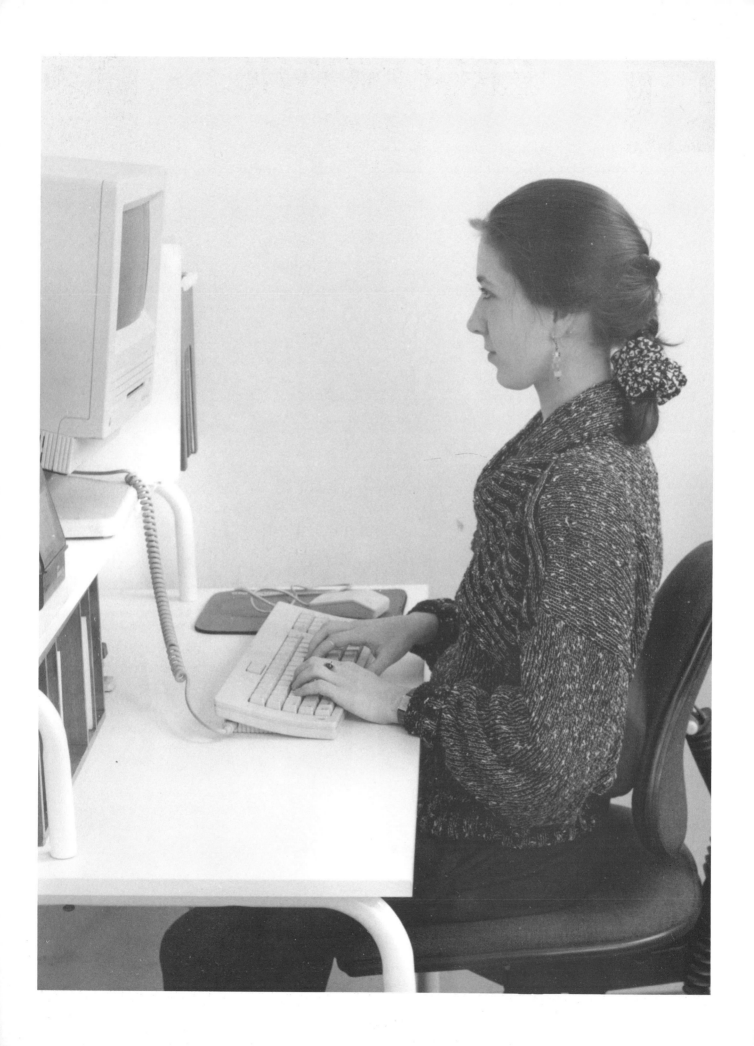

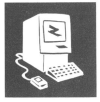

ERGONOMIC TIPS

George W., a thirty-four-year-old stockbroker, spent his entire work-day at a computer terminal or on the telephone. Though young and generally healthy, he was having aches and pains he thought more appropriate to someone fifty or sixty years old. When we talked with George, we discovered that he felt muscular discomfort only during the week and not at all on the weekends. We accompanied George to his workplace. After we showed George how to rearrange his computer terminal work area and gave him some basic ergonomic and sitting advice, he was able to work without suffering discomfort or pain any longer.

Ergonomics is a branch of engineering which seeks ways to improve conditions in the workplace in order to promote productivity, prevent injuries, and increase worker comfort.

Many muscular-skeletal aches and pains are associated with sedentary occupations and can be reduced with better ergonomic planning. Though we frequently tolerate working with uncomfortable chairs and desks, poor lighting, and improperly placed computer monitors, these are irritants, which often cause physical problems. This chapter and the previous chapter, "The Art of Dynamic Sitting," offer you effective commonsense techniques that can help improve the comfort of your work environment.

ERGONOMIC TIPS

CHAIRS

If you sit five hours a day or more, the type of chair you use is very important. Most office chairs offer inadequate support for your lower back and cause your lower back to round.

Well-designed chairs are becoming easier to find. They are known as ergonomic chairs and can provide excellent support for your lower back. No one chair is the right chair for everyone. There are many different styles and types of ergonomic chairs. The right chair for you will depend on the type of activities you do while seated, your body's structure and size, and any particular sensitivities you may have. Look for an ergonomic chair that has adjustable seat height and tilt, adjustable back height and tilt, adjustable armrests, and a contoured backrest that feels comfortable and allows you to change your position easily. If you don't have an ergonomic chair, we strongly recommend that you improve your chair by using a low back support or cushion. (See "The Art of Dynamic Sitting.")

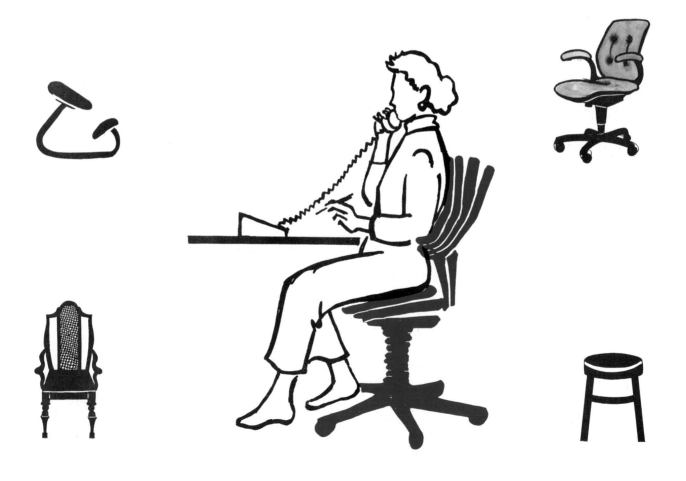

USING THE TELEPHONE

Holding a telephone for long periods of time can strain your neck, back, and shoulders. Every so often, switch the phone to your other ear. Speaker phones and headsets are two alternatives that can also reduce the physical strain of extensive telephone use.

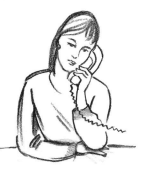

YOUR WORK SURFACE

The height of your desk or work surface may influence your comfort while you work. If your desk is too low, your back will become rounded, and the important natural arches of your spine will become diminished. If your desk is too high, your neck, shoulders, arms, and hands will become strained.

The right height for your work surface is determined by the sort of work you do and should allow you to sit efficiently and comfortably as described in "The Art of Dynamic Sitting." We recommend that you use a desk or work surface with adjustable height and tilt. This will allow you to adjust your work surface according to the type of work you are doing and reduce the need to lean forward. If your table is not adjustable, avoid leaning forward as much as possible.

TAKE BREAKS

We frequently neglect our physical comfort while we work, and forget about good sitting posture. To prevent a build-up of muscular tension and stress, it is a good idea to take short periodic breaks throughout the day. Even a very short break can make a big difference. If you have time, use Relaxercise for extra relief.

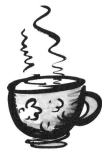

COMPUTER WORKSTATIONS

Millions of men and women spend their workday sitting in front of computer monitors or video display terminals (VDTs). VDT workers frequently suffer physical complaints, including back pain, neck and shoulder tension, and eye strain. VDT-related problems can be reduced, or in many cases eliminated, by following some simple ergonomic and health guidelines.

Use a well-designed ergonomic chair.

Sit close to your work surface.

Try to have the essential elements in your workstation —your chair, desk, monitor, keyboard, and work material— as mobile and adjustable as possible.

Your VDT screen should be fourteen to twenty-five inches from your eyes, depending on your visual acuity.

The center of your VDT screen should be level with your chin, or about ten degrees below your eye level.

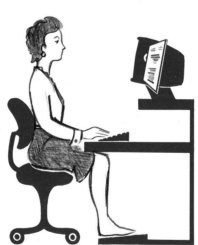

The height of your keyboard should permit your arms to slope downward slightly.

Your reference documents should be placed on an adjustable vertical stand next to your monitor so that you do not have to lean forward or change your focus.

Keep your work materials close to you.

Change your sitting position frequently.

Rest and exercise your hands and fingers whenever they feel strained or fatigued.

Periodically take a break and walk around or exercise. Try to take a significant break after every hour or two of VDT work.

Make your health and comfort a priority. When you feel good, you can work more efficiently and effectively.

VDT EYE CARE TIPS

- Your light source should not shine directly into your eyes or create glare or shadows. Natural light from a window is probably best. If you need artificial lighting, "full-spectrum" fluorescent light gives the most comfortable illumination.

- Close your eyes and rest them for a moment a few times during each hour of work.

- While working with a computer, the constant use of near vision is stressful to your eyes. To reduce the stress, take a moment every five to ten minutes to look away from your work, out a nearby window or around the room.

- When you look at a VDT monitor for a long period of time, your eyes remain relatively fixed and unmoving. This can impair your vision. To protect your eyes from damage and strain, frequently shift your gaze away from the screen.

- Use an antiglare, nonreflective screen over your monitor.

- Use a monitor with high resolution. These are easier to read and safer for your eyes.

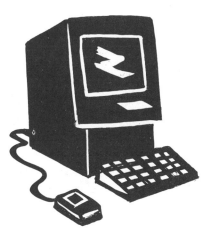

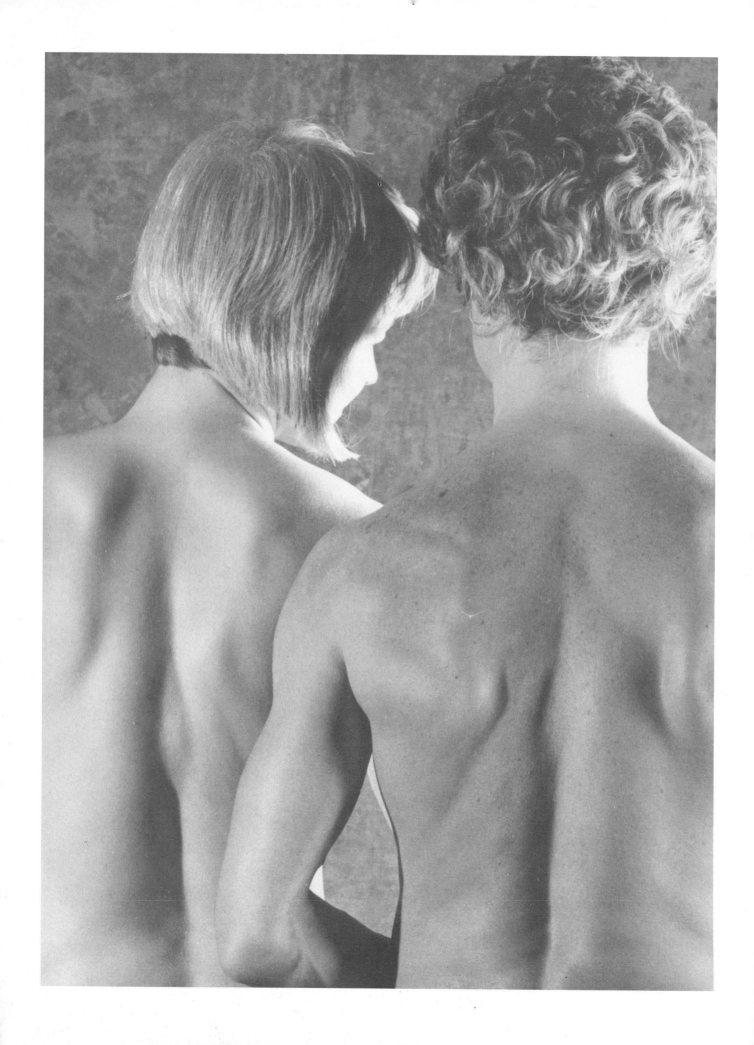

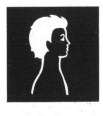

POSTURE TIPS

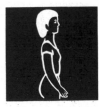

Norma P. came to us complaining of chronic shoulder pain and aching legs. As a young girl her parents frequently reminded her to sit up straight and all through her school years teachers admonished her for her poor posture. But what looked slouched or slumped over to others, felt natural and comfortable to Norma. Now, at the age of forty-six, she was feeling the consequences of a lifetime of unhealthy posture. We gave Norma a series of Relaxercise exercises to do at home and our guidelines for good sitting and standing posture. After three months her aches and pain had disappeared and when she was measured at the doctor's office, she had gained a full inch in height.

Good posture looks good and feels good. The old "stomach in, chest out, and shoulders back" routine is **not** good posture. Forcing your body into this uncomfortable and unnatural position creates muscular strain, fatigue, and discomfort. True good posture, on the other hand, actually relieves muscular tension, maximizes your energy, and allows you to move freely and efficiently.

When you use Relaxercise, your posture will improve automatically. This is because Relaxercise accesses the parts of your brain and nervous system that control your postural habits. Here are some additional tips to help you improve your posture. Remember that your sitting posture can be especially influential to your health and comfort. Information on sitting posture can be found in the chapter "The Art of Dynamic Sitting."

POSTURE TIPS

DYNAMIC STANDING POSTURE

- Stand with your feet about shoulder width apart. When your feet are too close together, your neck, back, and leg muscles tighten in order to maintain your balance. A wider base of support is always more stable and minimizes your body's muscular effort.

- Relax your knees. Locked knees restrict your hip joints and strain your back.

- Maintain the natural arches of your lower back and neck. These curves are absolutely essential for healthy posture.

- Wear comfortable, low-heeled shoes. High heels are bad for your posture because they tilt your weight too far forward and strain your back muscles. Wear shoes that have well-cushioned soles and provide good support.

- Reduce **all** unnecessary muscular effort in your body. In good posture, your skeleton, not your muscles, supports your body.

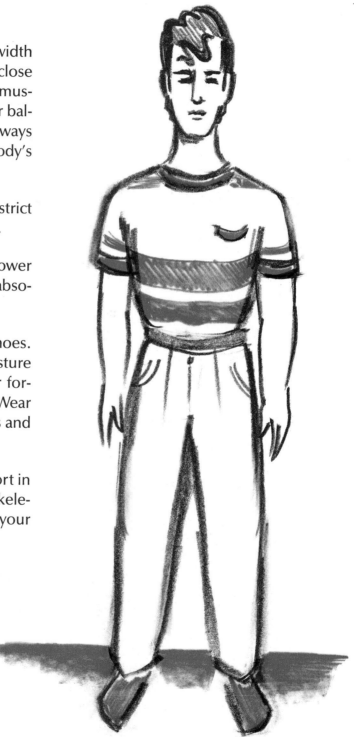

LIFTING SAFELY AND EASILY

One of the most common causes of serious back injury is the lifting of heavy objects, incorrectly. When you lift something from a bent-over position, the weight of the object becomes multiplied by a leverage factor of twelve to sixteen times. For example: when a 180-pound person lifts a 70-pound weight, he or she is exerting more than a thousand pounds of pressure on the discs of the lower back.

- Before you lift a heavy object, always spread your feet about shoulder width apart so you have a stable base of support.

- Stand close to the object you are intending to lift so that you will not have to lean or bend forward.

- Lower your body by bending your knees, while maintaining a slight arch of your lower back. This is very important.

- To lift the object, exhale while slowly straightening your legs. Let your legs and pelvis—not your back—do the work of lifting.

- Keep your neck and shoulders as relaxed as possible.

- If you intend to turn, wait until you have reached an upright position. Then carefully shift the weight of your pelvis and feet. Do not twist your back.

- While carrying a heavy object, minimize the pressure on your spine by maintaining your spine's natural curves and alignment.

CARRYING WEIGHT SAFELY

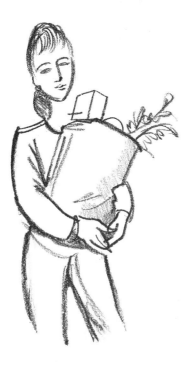

Whether you happen to be carrying a purse, briefcase, grocery bag, or baby, remember to share the work between both sides of your body. Always carrying weight with the same shoulder or arm can eventually cause serious muscular imbalances and tension throughout your body.

CAR SEATS

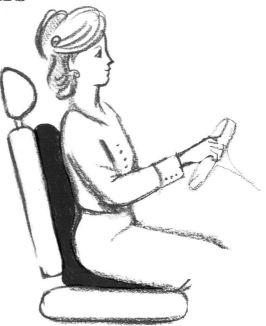

The seats in most cars and most forms of public transportation offer little or no support for your lower back. Some newer cars do have ergonomic seats that provide adjustable, low back support and seat-angle options.

If the seat of your car provides inadequate support for your back, it is worthwhile to use a low back support. (See "The Art of Dynamic Sitting.") Take one with you when you travel by plane or train. Special adjustable back supports made especially for car seats are available through orthopedic supply and back care stores. These provide a firm seat bottom and a contoured seat back.

SLEEPING

Sleeping in the same position night after night can create muscular imbalances and strain. Some health experts recommend a particular sleeping position, but unless you are in pain, it is a good idea to change and adjust your position freely whenever you like. If you suffer from acute back pain, you may find it helpful to sleep on your back or side with your knees slightly bent. When lying on your back, sleep with a pillow under your knees. When lying on your side, try sleeping with a pillow between your knees.

If you suffer from neck pain, your pillow may influence your nighttime comfort. Pillows that are too high or too low tend to overstretch your neck muscles. Pillows filled with goose or duck down are the most pliable variety of pillow and are easily shaped to suit your individual needs. There are also special orthopedic pillows available, which are shaped to support the arch of your neck.

Another common reason for nocturnal discomfort is sleeping on a mattress that is too soft. Studies of human sleep habits have shown that we move and change position frequently during the night. A very soft mattress can restrict your ability to turn and change position. A mattress that is firm, but not too hard, makes moving and changing your position during the night easier.

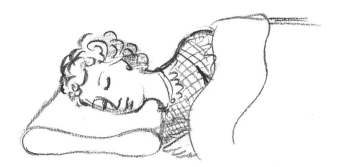

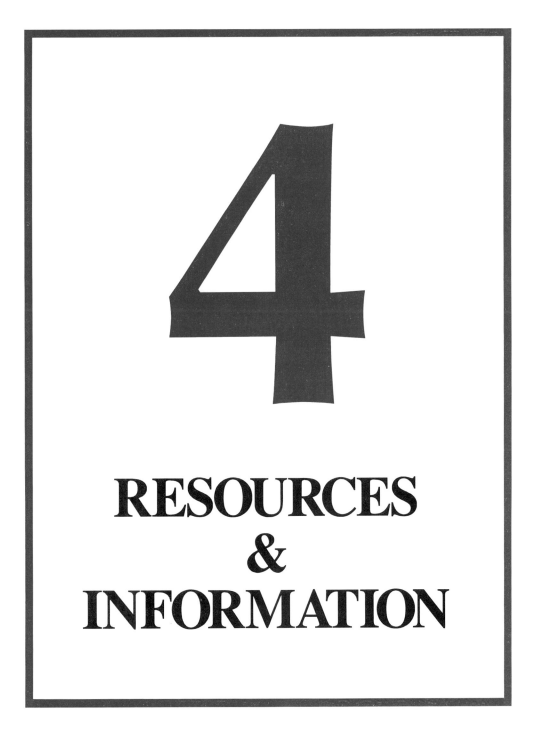

4

RESOURCES
&
INFORMATION

RESOURCE DIRECTORY

Relaxercise Audiotapes, Seminars, and Workshops

For information on specialized programs and products created by the authors of this book for the public and health professionals, write to:

Sensory Motor Learning Systems
P.O. Box 5674
Berkeley, Calif. 94705

Feldenkrais Method Teachers

For a listing of authorized Feldenkrais Teachers in North America, write to: S.M.L.S. or,

Feldenkrais Guild of North America
14 Corporate Woods
8717 West 110th Street, Suite 140
Overland Park, Kans. 66210

Back Comfort Stores

The following specialized retail stores sell state-of-the-art ergonomic chairs, tables, car seats, beds, and other accessories for people wanting to be more comfortable and for those with serious back problems. This is only a partial listing. For a store in your area, consult your phone directory under "orthopedic supplies" or call one of the following stores for a referral.

Back Care Shop
10475 Montgomery Road
Cincinnati, Ohio 45242
(513) 793-7335

Back Designs
614 Grand Avenue
Oakland, Calif. 94610
(415) 451-6600
(Publishes an impressive
direct mail catalog.)

Back Relief and Comfort Store
2112 Highway 35
Ocean, N.J. 07712
(201) 493-BACK

Back Store
2111 Yonge Street
Toronto, Ontario
Canada M4S2A4
(416) 482-0771

Better Back Store
3333 South Wadsworth Blvd.
#C107
Lakewood, Colo. 80227
(303) 980-6860

Sensible Seating
4308 Montgomery Avenue
Bethesda, Md. 20814
(301) 652-7788

REFERENCES AND SUGGESTED READINGS

Books by Moshe Feldenkrais

Body and Mature Behavior: A Study of Anxiety, Sex, Gravitation, and Learning. New York: International Universities Press, 1950.

Awareness Through Movement: Health Exercises for Personal Growth. New York: Harper & Row, 1972.

The Case of Nora. New York: Harper & Row, 1977.

The Elusive Obvious. Cupertino, Calif.: Meta Publications, 1981.

The Master Moves. Cupertino, Calif.: Meta Publications, 1984.

The Potent Self. New York: Harper & Row, 1985.

Books about the Feldenkrais Method

Hanna, Thomas. *The Body of Life.* New York: Knopf, 1980.

Masters, Robert, and Jean Houston. *Listening to the Body.* New York: Delacorte Press, 1978.

Rywerant, Yochanan. *The Feldenkrais Method.* San Francisco: Harper & Row, 1983.

Anatomy and Kinesics

Broer, Marion R. *An Introduction to Kinesiology.* Englewood Cliffs, N.J.: Prentice-Hall, 1968.

————. *Efficiency of Human Movement.* Philadelphia: Saunders, 1967.

Kapanji, I. A. *Physiology of the Joints.* 3 vols. New York: Churchill, 1982.

Kapit, Wynn, and Lawrence Elson. *The Anatomy Coloring Book.* New York: Harper & Row, 1977.

The Brain

Brown, Barbara. *New Mind, New Body.* New York: Irvington, 1986.

Green, Elmer, and Alyce Green. *Beyond Biofeedback.* New York: Delacorte Press, 1977.

Ornstein, Robert, Richard Thompson, and David Macaulay. *The Amazing Brain.* Boston: Houghton Mifflin, 1984.

Pribram, Karl. *Languages of the Brain.* Englewood Cliffs, N.J.: Prentice-Hall, 1971.

Restak, Richard M. *The Brain.* New York: Doubleday, 1979.

Sacks, Oliver. *The Man Who Mistook His Wife for a Hat.* New York: Summit Books, 1985.

Illness and Healing

Bresler, David E., with Richard Trubo. *Free Yourself from Pain*. New York: Simon & Schuster, 1979.

Cailliet, René. *Soft Tissue, Pain and Disability*. 2nd ed. Philadelphia: Davis, 1988.

Cousins, Norman. *Anatomy of an Illness*. New York: Norton, 1979.

Jaffe, Dennis T. *Healing from Within*. New York: Simon & Schuster, 1988.

Miller, Emmett. *Self-Imagery: Creating Your Own Good Health*. Rev. ed. Berkeley, Calif.: Celestial Arts, 1986.

Ornstein, Robert, and David Sobel. *The Healing Brain*. New York: Simon & Schuster, 1987.

Pelletier, Kenneth R. *Mind as Healer, Mind as Slayer*. New York: Delta, 1977.

Rossi, Ernest L. *Psychobiology of Mind-Body Healing: New Concepts of Therapeutic Hypnosis*. New York: Norton, 1988.

Rossi, Ernest, and David B. Cheek. *Mind-Body Therapy*. New York: Norton, 1988.

Rossman, Martin L. *Healing Yourself*. New York: Walker & Co., 1987.

Sacks, Oliver. *A Leg to Stand On*. New York: Harper & Row, 1984.

Sarno, John. *Mind over Back Pain*. New York: Morrow, 1984.

Siegel, Bernie S. *Love, Medicine and Miracles*. New York: Harper & Row, 1986.

Simonton, Carl, Stephanie Matthews-Simonton, and James Creighton. *Getting Well Again*. New York: Bantam, 1982.

Relaxation and Stress Reduction

Benson, Herbert. *The Relaxation Response*. New York: Morrow, 1975.

———. *Beyond the Relaxation Response*. New York: Times Books, 1984.

Davis, Martha, Elizabeth Robbins Eshelman, and Mathew McKay. *The Relaxation and Stress Reduction Workbook*. Oakland, Calif.: New Harbinger Publications, 1988.

Dychtwald, Ken. *Bodymind*. New York: Jove, 1977.

Goleman, Daniel, and Tara Bennett-Goleman. *The Relaxed Body Book*. Garden City, N.Y.: Doubleday, 1986.

Stransky, Judith, with Robert B. Stone. *The Alexander Technique*. New York: Beaufort Books, 1981.

Music Education

Chase, Mildred Portney. *Just Being at the Piano*. Peace Press, 1974.

Ristad, Eloise. *A Soprano on Her Head*. Moab, Utah: Real People Press, 1982.

Wilson, Frank R. *Tone Deaf and All Thumbs*. New York: Random House, 1987.

Sports and Fitness

Blanchard, Kenneth, D. W. Eddington, and Marjorie Blanchard. *The One-Minute Manager Gets Fit*. New York: Morrow, 1986.

Gallwey, Timothy W. *Inner Tennis*. New York: Bantam, 1979.

Heggie, Jack. *Running with the Whole Body*. Emmaus, Pa.: Rodale Press, 1986.

Murphy, Michael. *Golf in the Kingdom*. New York: Dell, 1973.

Solomon, Henry. *The Exercise Myth*. New York: Bantam, 1984.

Science and Philosophy

Bateson, Gregory. *Mind and Nature*. New York: Dutton, 1979.

Capra, Fritjof. *The Tao of Physics*. Boston: Shambhala, 1975.

————. *The Turning Point: Science, Society and the Rising Culture*. New York: Simon & Schuster, 1982.

Wilber, Ken, ed. *Holographic Paradigm and Other Paradoxes*. Boston: Shambhala, 1982.

Psychology and Learning

Bloomfield, Harold, and Robert B. Kory. *Inner Joy*. New York: Jove, 1985.

Bry, Adelaide. *Visualization*. New York: Barnes & Noble, 1978.

DeBono, Edward. *Lateral Thinking*. New York: Harper & Row, 1970.

Gawain, Shakti. *Creative Visualization*. New York: Bantam, 1982.

Gendlin, Eugene. *Focusing*. New York: Bantam, 1981.

Gilligan, Stephen G. *Therapeutic Trances*. New York: Brunner/Mazel, 1987.

Grinder, John, and Richard Bandler. *TRANCE-formations*. Moab, Utah: Real People Press, 1985.

Hofstadter, Douglas R., and Daniel C. Dennett. *The Mind's I*. New York: Basic Books, 1981.

Keen, Sam. *To a Dancing God*. New York: Harper & Row, 1970.

Ostrander, Sheila, and Lynn Schroeder. *Superlearning*. New York: Dell, 1980.

Reese, Mark. "Moshe Feldenkrais's Work with Movement: A Parallel Approach to Milton Erickson's Hypnotherapy." In *Ericksonian Psychotherapy*, vol. 1, edited by J. Zeig. New York: Brunner/Mazel, 1985.

————. "Moshe Feldenkrais's Verbal Approach to Somatic Education: Parallels to Milton Erickson's Use of Language." In *Hypnotic and Strategic Interventions*, edited by Michael D. Yapko. New York: Irvington, 1986.

Schutz, Will. *Profound Simplicity*. New York: Bantam, 1979.

Smith, Adam. *Powers of Mind*. New York: Random House, 1975.

Zeig, J. K., ed. *A Teaching Seminar with Milton Erickson, M.D.* New York: Brunner/Mazel, 1980.

INDEX

THE AUTHORS

David Zemach-Bersin, Ph.D., and Mark Reese, Ph.D., are co-founders of Sensory Motor Learning Systems and creators of the Relaxercise system. They present workshops and lead specialized training programs for health professionals and businesses throughout the world.

Dr. Zemach-Bersin is former president of the Feldenkrais Guild of North America. He and his wife Kaethe, and three daughters live in Berkeley, California, where he teaches and conducts a private practice.

Dr. Reese has published numerous articles on health and psychology. He and his wife Donna, and two children live in San Diego, California, where he conducts a private practice in the Feldenkrais Method.

Kaethe Zemach-Bersin is the designer, illustrator, and co-author of *Relaxercise*. She lives in Berkeley, California, with her husband and daughters.

Sensory Motor Learning Systems, founded in 1983, produces innovative health, fitness, and movement improvement programs for health professionals, business, hospitals, and the general public. Specialized programs and products have been created to meet the needs of athletes, sedentary workers, people with neuromuscular problems, the elderly, and the disabled.